# Dedication

To our families
for their support

To our teachers
for their wisdom

To our students
for their direction

To our patients
for their trust

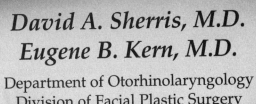

**David A. Sherris, M.D.**
**Eugene B. Kern, M.D.**

Department of Otorhinolaryngology
Division of Facial Plastic Surgery
Mayo Clinic
Rochester, Minnesota

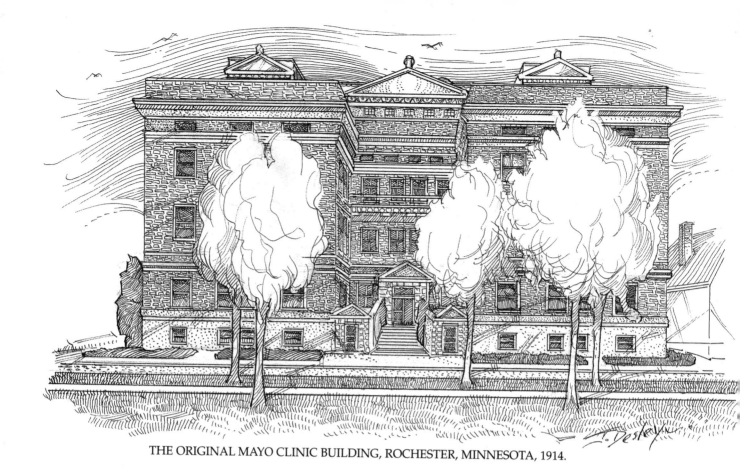

THE ORIGINAL MAYO CLINIC BUILDING, ROCHESTER, MINNESOTA, 1914.

The triple-shield Mayo logo and the words MAYO, MAYO CLINIC, and MAYO CLINIC SCIENTIFIC PRESS are marks of Mayo Foundation for Medical Education and Research.

© 1999 Mayo Foundation for Medical Education and Research

All rights are reserved. This book is protected by copyright. No part of it may be reproduced, stored in a retrieval system, or transmitted, in any form or by any means--electronic, mechanical, photocopying, recording, or otherwise--without the prior written consent of the copyright holder, except for brief quotations embodied in critical articles and reviews. Inquiries should be addressed to Mayo Clinic, 200 First Street SW, Rochester, MN 55905.

Care has been taken to confirm the accuracy of the information presented and to describe generally accepted practices. However, the authors, editor, and publisher are not responsible for errors or omissions or for any consequences from application of the information in this book and make no warranty, express or implied, with respect to the contents of the publication.

The authors, editor, and publisher have exerted efforts to ensure that drug selection and dosage set forth in this text are in accordance with current recommendations and practice at the time of publication. However, in view of ongoing research, changes in government regulations, and the constant flow of information relating to drug therapy and drug reactions, the reader is urged to check the package insert for each drug for any change in indications and dosage and for added warnings and precautions. This is particularly important when the recommended agent is a new or infrequently employed drug.

Some drugs and medical devices presented in this publication have Food and Drug Administration (FDA) clearance for limited use in restricted research settings. It is the responsibility of the health care providers to ascertain the FDA status of each drug or device planned for use in their clinical practice.

ISBN 1-893005-51-8

# Preface

The current education for medical students in the realm of surgery has been markedly compacted; often the allotted time in which the principles of surgery must be taught and learned does not extend beyond six weeks. This adverse situation is compounded by the reduced time that the surgical faculty spends with students. The same socioeconomic forces that have caused this behavior pattern also account for the reduction of time during which the surgical faculty formally educates. Sadly, basic principles have been poorly addressed. Residency Review Committees concerned with this circumstance have mandated exposure of surgical residents to basic science as it pertains to surgery. This is certainly appropriate but it is equally appropriate to stress basic technical principles of operative procedures because the technical therapies are uniquely in the surgeon's armamentarium. The ability to treat by an operation distinguishes the surgeon from the physician.

In learning the principles of surgery, the principles of technique constitute an essential ingredient. This ingredient has been neglected recently. The authors of Basic Surgical Skills have filled a void. They have provided in a succinct, readable, and understandable text the bases of surgical techniques. The CD-ROM elegantly clarifies the written words. The audience should include all medical students as they rotate through their exposure to surgery and all residents in surgical specialties as they launch their training programs. The word "education" derives from the Latin, meaning "lead out." The combined words and views serve to lead the novitiates in the field of surgery into the surgical arena, the operating room. ■

Seymour I. Schwartz, M.D., F.A.C.S.*

Professor of Surgery

University of Rochester School of Medicine and Dentistry

Rochester, New York

*Corbett*

* F.A.C.S. - Fellow, American College of Surgeons, past president of the American College of Surgeons

# Contents

# Introduction

So you want to work in surgery! This manual (with CD ROM) is for beginners. As a beginner, you must learn the basic technical skills necessary if you wish to become a competent surgeon or surgical assistant. This program is designed to present the materials in a user-friendly manner. Thus, the surgical scrub, anesthetics, infiltration techniques, basic instruments, incisions, wound closures, suture material, knot tying, basic soft tissue flaps, the fundamentals of tissue injury, wound healing and general postoperative care will all be covered in this manual. We want you to learn to perform basic maneuvers fundamental to all surgery. We are not teaching the medicine of surgery. Thus the details of surgical judgment or specific problems related to, for example, general, orthopedic, cardiac, or other forms of surgery are just beyond the scope of this work. We have designed the manual to be visual and concise to speed the learning process. The text is brief. The drawings and photographs are numerous and, we hope, all-inclusive. We have prepared a glossary of terms. The words that are underlined in the text are defined in the glossary. For example, **surgery** is underlined in the text, so it appears in the glossary.

We have designed the CD ROM portion to review the basics and supplement the manual with execution of exercises in both animated and live filmed video presentations.

CD ROM icon indicates supplemental audio-visual materials that can be seen on the CD.

You will practice all the basic surgical techniques on pigs' feet. In addition, there will be tests of your knowledge. Knowledge of surgical ideas and technical experience on pigs' feet will make you self-assured. Being self-assured in the operating room is a great feeling! So, on your mark, get set, let's go and begin to learn the basic surgical skills so you can stride into the operating room with knowledge, experience, and confidence.

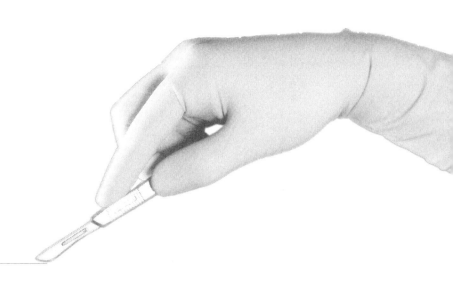

# A. The Operating Room

The operating room is a special and unique place. The personnel are trained for their specific jobs and routines.

**Anesthesiologists** and **nurse anesthetists** are an important part of the surgical team. They are responsible for the anesthetic care of the surgical patient whether surgery is performed under general **intubation** anesthesia, attended local anesthesia, or local anesthesia.

During general intubation anesthesia, the patient is totally asleep. Under attended local anesthesia, the patient is awake but receiving some type of sedation. Under local anesthesia alone the patient is not sedated, and monitoring is less essential. The vital signs, blood pressure, pulse, **oxygen saturation**, and **electrocardiogram** are all monitored by the anesthesia team. The surgical "scrub" nurse (gowned and gloved in a **sterile** manner) is responsible for the set-up of the surgical instruments. The "scrub" nurse also helps direct the operating room activities in an orderly and efficient manner. The "circulating nurse" is also in attendance. This individual is unscrubbed and unsterile and is helpful in obtaining various materials when needed during the surgery. He/she also assists in taking specimens to **pathology**, answering pagers and telephone calls, and various other activities as they arise during the surgical procedure. Obviously, the surgeon and surgical assistants are also an integral part of the surgical team.

The operating room atmosphere should be one of professionalism — warm, friendly, caring and efficient. Frequently music is played in order to provide a sense of relaxation to the environment. There are times when a situation in the operating room can be tense. It takes practice and discipline for the many personality types who are in the operating room to maintain their cool during the stress of an operation. Loss of control can be demeaning to the staff in an operating room setting and has no place in the professional surgical environment. There are times, however, when a situation becomes so stressful that control is difficult. Words may be said in frustration or anger. It's never too late to apologize. The entire team is present to help the surgeon and surgical assistants accomplish the task for the welfare of the patient. Maintain your cool, become a teacher, and the golden rule is certainly applicable here. Treat people the way you would like to be treated. It's a great and rare privilege to be involved in the miracle of health restored. The operating room is a place where that miracle frequently unfolds.

# B. The Wound

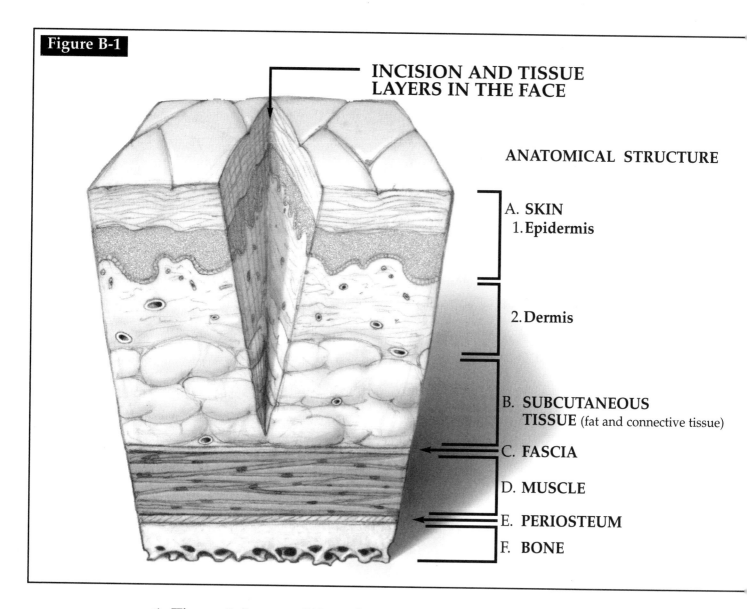

**Figure B-1**

### INCISION AND TISSUE LAYERS IN THE FACE

**ANATOMICAL STRUCTURE**

A. **SKIN**
   1. Epidermis

   2. Dermis

B. **SUBCUTANEOUS TISSUE** (fat and connective tissue)

C. **FASCIA**

D. **MUSCLE**

E. **PERIOSTEUM**

F. **BONE**

## 1. Tissue Injury — Wounding

There are three distinct stages of tissue injury (wounding) and repair (healing). These include: 1) inflammation; 2) proliferation and scar formation; and 3) maturation. **Figure B-1** is a wound created by incision in the face. Be able to list all components included in the tissue layers.

### a. Inflammation, stage 1 (1-5 days)

After the initial tissue injury, the inflammatory response produced by the tissues involves a diffuse increase in tissue fluids. In addition, there is an increase in blood sup-ply and cellular elements (which appear in damaged tissue). This occurs in order to begin the healing or repair process. The increased blood supply causes **erythematous** skin changes. During this phase, **lymphocytes** and other cellular elements remove damaged and dead tissue by the action of the **enzymes** (**Figure B-2**). This removal of damaged tissue is termed "debridement." This action of **"debridement"** is produced by the proteolytic enzyme activity of the white blood cells (**leukocytes**). Pain is a normal protective response to tissue injury.

# B. The Wound

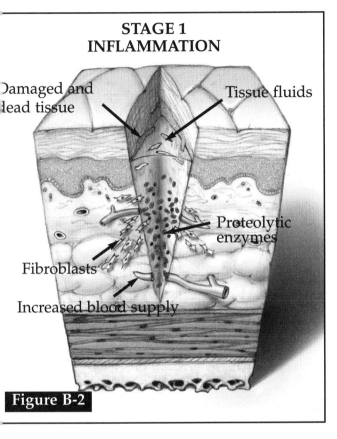

## STAGE 1
## INFLAMMATION

Damaged and dead tissue

Tissue fluids

Proteolytic enzymes

Fibroblasts

Increased blood supply

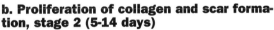

**Figure B-2**

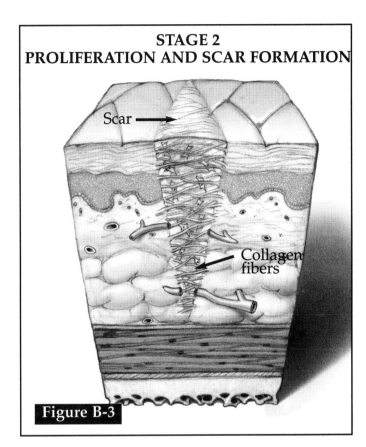

## STAGE 2
## PROLIFERATION AND SCAR FORMATION

Scar

Collagen fibers

**Figure B-3**

**b. Proliferation of collagen and scar formation, stage 2 (5-14 days)**

**Fibroblasts** produce the **collagen** fibers which are dispensed into the wound. The major substance of connective tissue is collagen. It is the collagen that helps determine the tensile strength of the wound and produces the scar (**cicatrix**) **(Figure B-3)**.

**c. Scar maturation, stage 3 (14 days – final healing)**

During the scar maturation stage, a significant amount of collagen is produced, dispensed, and remodeled across the wounded tissues. After a period of time, the wound can withstand normal stress. In addition, the scar usually contracts during this phase. The duration of this phase is variable, depending on the specific type of tissues that are wounded **(Figure B-4)**. About 95% of the full strength of the wound is usually reached by six weeks after injury.

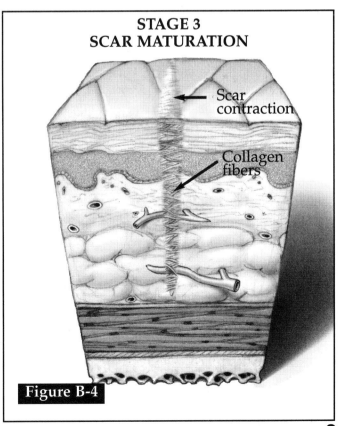

## STAGE 3
## SCAR MATURATION

Scar contraction

Collagen fibers

**Figure B-4**

9

# B. The Wound

## 2. Wound Classification

Wounds are classified according to the estimate of bacterial contamination and the possible risk of infection. Wound classification includes four types of wounds.

### a. Clean wounds

Most wounds created in surgery are made in a sterile environment and are rarely infected. Incision and wound closure using sutures is termed "closure by primary intention." Primary intention is the method of choice for closing a wound. This type of closure carries minimal risk of postoperative complications, since the surgery is performed under sterile conditions.

### b. Clean contaminated wounds

If during the course of an operation a muccus membrane lined cavity is entered, you have a clean wound that is now contaminated. For example, if the oral pharyngeal cavity (upper aerodigestive tract), genitourinary (GU), or gastrointestinal (GI) tract is entered, then you have a wound that was initially clean but is now contaminated by virtue of entry into a field contaminated with bacteria. A common operation, appendectomy, is an example of a clean contaminated wound.

### c. Contaminated wounds

Contaminated wounds are wounds in whic there is already exposure to microorganism Examples of contaminated wounds are trau matic injuries, open fractures, or entry into the genitourinary tract (GU), the gastrointestinal (GI) tract, or biliary tract. These co taminated wounds may become infected.

### d. Infected wounds

Infected wounds are also called "dirty" wounds because they are already growing bacteria, and pus has developed. They are clinically infected before surgery is performed. For example, an abscess is an infected wound. Wounds with **devitalized** or dying tissue are also already infected. Infection at the time of operation can increase the postoperative complication rat considerably.

# B. The Wound

## 3. Factors That Affect Wound Healing

You need to know those factors which are basic to all operative procedures that may affect both the results of the surgery and well-being of the patient.

### a. Age
The patient's age may affect wound healing. Children tend to heal with a robust response and may get **hypertrophic scars**. As the years pass, metabolic changes occur that are associated with both vascular insufficiencies and a lack of tissue elasticity. Because of these factors, old age may prolong or delay the healing of a wound.

### b. Weight
Excessive fat may prevent adequate wound closure. Fat itself has a reduced blood supply and, therefore, makes the patient vulnerable to infection and/or a delay in healing.

### c. Nutrition
Proteins, vitamins, and adequate hydration are all necessary to promote wound healing. Deficiencies in any of these important elements may disturb and delay wound healing.

### d. Dehydration
Adequate **electrolyte** balance and fluid levels are crucial to both kidney and cardiac function. The basic **metabolic** processes of the body require proper fluid balance to promote wound healing.

### e. Blood supply
Adequate blood supply to the wound site is necessary to promote wound healing. Poor circulation, diabetes, or other vascular illnesses may diminish the blood supply to the wound and can result in a delay in healing.

### f. Immune responses
**Immune** response deficiencies may significantly compromise surgical procedures. Patients who have **HIV**, who have been on high dosages of steroids for a prolonged period of time or who have had chemotherapy may have a deficient immune response. These factors may interfere with and delay the healing process.

### g. Chronic illness
Patients who have concomitant systemic illness or **endocrine** disorders such as diabetes are more likely to have postoperative complications with prolonged or delayed healing. Other situations involving systemic illness, including malignancies, may complicate wound healing.

### h. Drugs and radiation therapy
Steroids, immunosuppressive drugs, **antineoplastic** drugs, or **radiation therapy** may significantly disturb and delay wound healing.

### i. Smoking
Smoking can cause lung complications and it can prolong and disturb wound healing. Patients who do smoke should stop one week before surgery to prevent complications. Smoking ideally should be totally terminated.

# B. The Wound

## 4. Healing

Fundamentally there are three types or methods of healing.

### a. Primary intention

As mentioned, healing by primary intention is that which follows surgical wound closure with sutures. Uncomplicated healing by primary intention occurs with minimal edema, minimal discharge, and no bacterial infection. The tensile strength of the wound increases significantly, and the skin obtains approximately 85-90% of its tensile strength before the wounding. Healing by primary intention is the most desirable to the surgeon.

### b. Secondary intention

If the healing does not occur by primary intention and the wound is left to granulate closed, this is termed healing by secondary intention. Healing by secondary intention occurs when the wound is left open and the healing proceeds with **granulation tissue** from the deeper layers out toward the surface of the skin. Healing by secondary intention is a slower process and usually takes four to eight weeks to re-epithelialize the area.

### c. Tertiary intention

This is also termed delayed primary closure. This is the method of choice in contaminated, dirty, infected wounds with loss of tissue. The surgeon may debride the nonviable tissue before closure. Surgical closure with sutures is usually performed about four to six days after injury. Unlike secondary intention, the wound is closed with delayed suturing, rather than being allowed to close entirely by granulation.

### d. Complications

Significant problems that complicate healing are: infection, wound breakdown (**dehiscence**), **hematoma**, **seroma**, **hypertrophic scars** and **keloids**. Organisms that find their way into the wound may produce delayed healing, generalized **bacteremia**, **gangrene**, or even death. Antibiotics alone may be used when **cellulitis** occurs. If abscess or **necrosis** occurs, the wound must first be incised and drained with removal (**debridement**) of dead tissue before healing can occur. Wound **dehiscence** may occur in areas prone to movement, in elderly patients, in the debilitated, or can result from inappropriate or improper suture techniques.

A **hematoma** is a collection of blood in the depths of a wound, while a seroma is a collection of serous fluid in the depths of a wound. Hematomas usually result from inadequate **hemostasis** at surgery, or reopening of a blood vessel after surgery. Some factors predisposing to hematoma formation include hypertension, bleeding disorders and presence of excessive dead space in a wound. Untreated, hematomas may lead to abscess formation, loss of skin (slough), or excessive scar tissue. When recognized, hematomas must be treated expeditiously by reopening and draining the blood.

**Seroma** is a collection of **serum** in the tissues and usually occurs later in the wound healing process. This is a result of dead space in a wound or excessive movement of tissues (i.e., muscles) under a wound which allows fluid devoid of red blood cells to collect. The risk of seroma formation can be decreased by careful closure of all of the layers of the wound and by immobilizing the wound during the healing phase. Close all dead spaces. If they occur, seromas should also be drained to prevent further complications. Sometimes this can be done with a needle and syringe, while other times the wound must be reopened.

**Hypertrophic scars** and **keloids** are erythematous, tender, elevated, unsightly scars that may itch or produce a contraction cicatrix. The clinical difference between the two is that a keloid extends beyond the margins of the initial scar while a hypertrophic scar does not. Many treatments are available for each and include surgical scar revision, pressure dressings, and steroid injections. Further discussion of these entities is beyond the scope of this work.

# *Quiz*

Fill in the shaded blanks! See page 8, Figure B-1 for the correct answers.

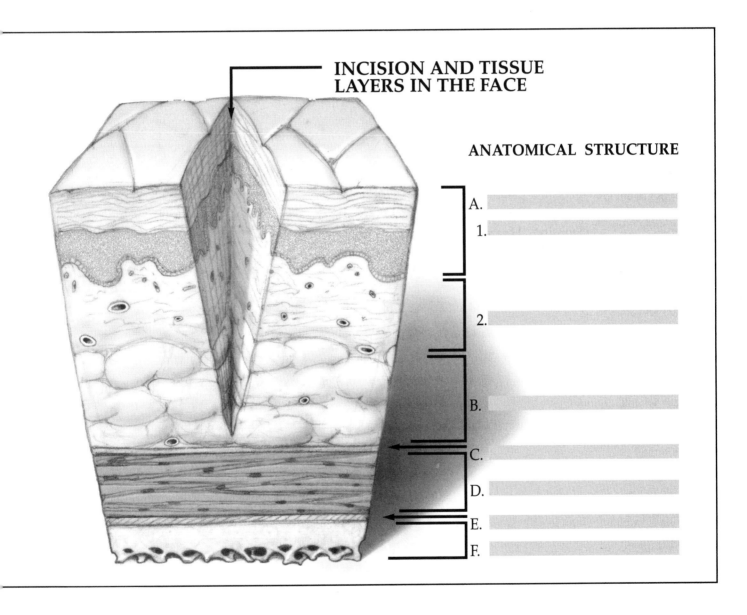

**INCISION AND TISSUE LAYERS IN THE FACE**

**ANATOMICAL STRUCTURE**

A.

1.

2.

B.

C.

D.

E.

F.

# C. Basic Principles in Surgery

There are a number of basic surgical principles that you must be aware of when performing surgery.

## 1. Hemostasis

Bleeding is the enemy of proper visualization (exposure) during surgery. If you can't see, you can't operate safely. A "dry" (bloodless) surgical field is crucial for adequate visualization. In addition, when the surgical field is dry, the accumulation of serum or blood is minimal. If blood does accumulate in the wound after the surgical procedure is finished, this is termed a hematoma. Hematoma can lead to infection or to a delay in wound healing. It must be drained.

## 2. Handling of the Tissues

Be gentle to the tissues. Use a dissection technique that produces minimal tissue trauma. It is also crucial to preserve all vital structures including nerves, blood vessels (arteries and veins), connective tissue, and muscles. Retraction (pulling on the tissues) should be firm yet gentle since injury to tissues can impair wound healing and allow bacteria to colonize.

## 3. Incision Planning

Why do we incise the skin? Actually, surgeons make incisions for a variety of reasons. The reasons include excision (surgical removal) of skin lesions, exposure of deeper structures for other surgical procedures, and reconstruction of traumatic defects. Yet, prior to making any incision, planning is necessary. As the surgeon, you must choose an incision that will accomplish several goals. First, the incision chosen must result in the best scar. The best scar is the least noticeable and has the least interference with function. A well-planned incision will allow you to adequately expose the underlying structures and avoid injury to critical deeper structures like major nerves, arteries, veins, and vital organs.

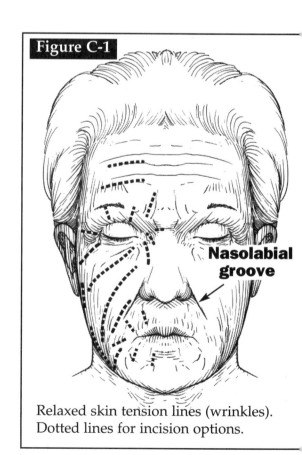

**Figure C-1**

**Nasolabial groove**

Relaxed skin tension lines (wrinkles). Dotted lines for incision options.

# C. Basic Principles in Surgery

Figure C-2

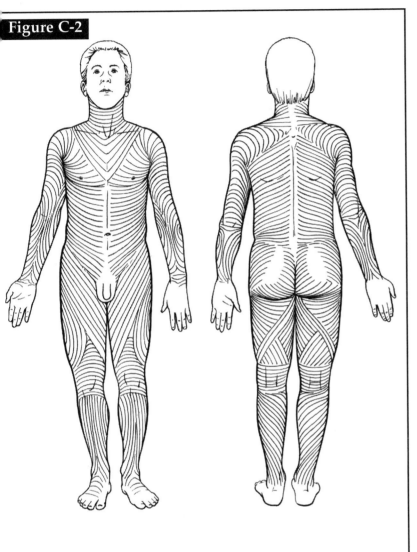

Relaxed skin tension lines — Lines for incision placement.

## 4. Relaxed Skin Tension Lines

A good scar results when the skin incisions are made along the lines (axis) of the relaxed skin tension lines (**Figure C-1, C-2**). Relaxed skin tension lines are the lines of minimal tension of the skin. Incisions should be made on or parallel to these lines so that they are under the least possible tension while healing and produce a minimal scar. The technique used in the incision itself and the amount of wound closing tension are also critical things to consider in order to produce a minimal or less noticeable scar.

As far as the incision itself, it needs to be planned well before a knife is utilized — thus the dictum **"decision before incision."**

Incisions parallel to relaxed skin tension lines along aesthetic unit boundaries and in the midline of the face and body heal with less perceptible scarring. The aesthetic boundaries include things like the cheek and the lip boundary (the nasolabial groove) and the border of the eyebrow where there are natural shadows and contour changes to help camouflage or hide the scar.

As far as the incision itself is concerned, the scalpel should be used to make a skin cut perpendicular to the skin edge and not **beveled**. In rare circumstances, the surgeon intentionally bevels the skin edge. A beveled edge is usually more difficult to close surgically with good apposition of the wound edges. The incision perpendicular to the skin edge is easier to get good apposition of the wound edges which results in a better (less noticeable) scar.

## 5. Undermining

After incision or excision, undermining (relaxing or loosening) of the skin edges surrounding the defect assists in wound closure (**Figure C-3, 1-7**). This is because the wound edges can be brought together under less tension by combining both deep (subcutaneous or subcuticular) sutures and skin sutures. Also, the act of undermining itself relaxes the skin so that it is under less tension.

# C. Basic Principles in Surgery

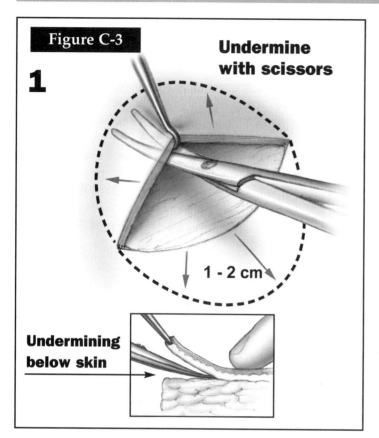

**Figure C-3**

**1**

**Undermine with scissors**

1 - 2 cm

**Undermining below skin**

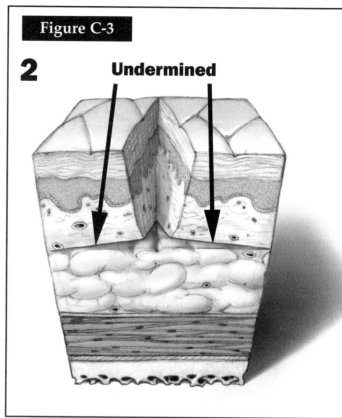

**Figure C-3**

**2**

**Undermined**

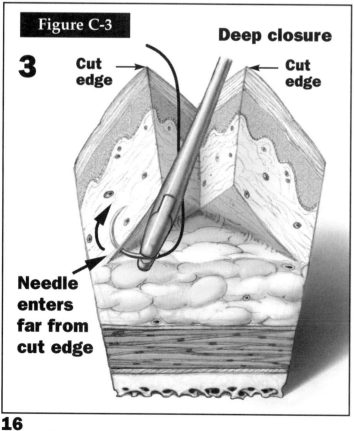

**Figure C-3**

**3**

**Deep closure**

Cut edge

Cut edge

**Needle enters far from cut edge**

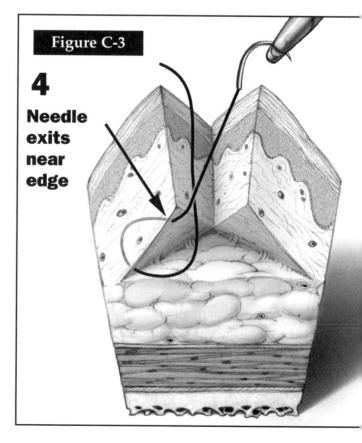

**Figure C-3**

**4**

**Needle exits near edge**

# C. Basic Principles in Surgery

**Figure C-3**

**5**

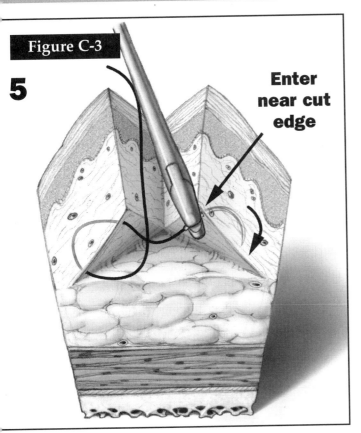

**Enter near cut edge**

**Figure C-3**

**6**

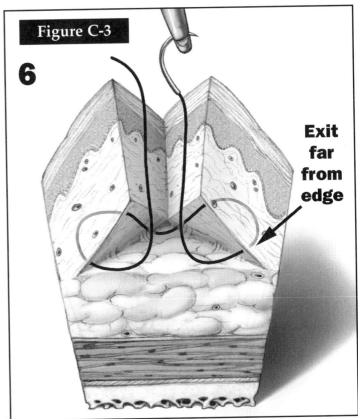

**Exit far from edge**

**Figure C-3**

**7**

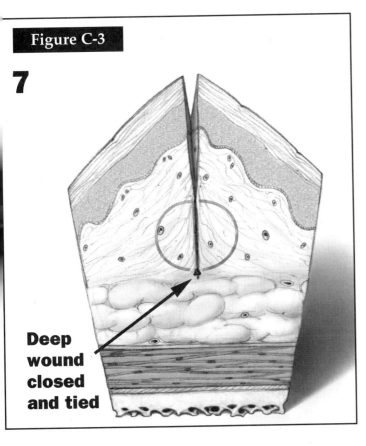

**Deep wound closed and tied**

# C. Basic Principles in Surgery

## 6. Choice of Suture Materials

The proper suture material is required so that the tissues in each layer can be adequately approximated (*See SECTION G, Sutures and Knots pgs. 42-76*). Suture materials maximize healing by approximating the tissues being operated on. The reaction of the body to various suture materials may be either minimal or intense. Intense tissue reaction involves swelling (edema) that can delay healing. Careful and precise suture placement, with the proper amount of tension, promotes healing.

## 7. Closing With Sufficient Tension

It is important to approximate the wound, which means to bring the edges of the wound in close proximity to each other, but not too tightly. The dictum **"approximate, don't strangulate"** guides the surgeon during closure. You will learn the feel of the proper amount of tension required to close a wound. Excessive tissue tension or tissue strangulation can also be uncomfortable to the patient and may lead to infection and delayed healing.

## 8. Tissue Moisture

Long procedures may require periodic lavage (washing) of the operative field with warm saline to prevent drying of tissue.

## 9. Debriding Necrotic (Dead) Tissue

All **devitalized** (necrotic) tissue needs to be removed so that healing can occur, especially in traumatized wounds. For example, foreign bodies, including road debris, dirt, glass, and wood fragments, need to be debrided before you close the wound so the possibility of infection is markedly reduced.

# C. Basic Principles in Surgery

## 10. Dead Spaces

Dead spaces are areas in the wound that have not been adequately closed. It is important that each layer be closed individually, especially in the fatty layers. Dead space facilitates wound separation, seroma or hematoma formation, and bacterial overgrowth **(Figure C-3, #8)**. It may be necessary to either apply a pressure dressing or insert a drain (or both) to help eliminate dead space even after adequate closure of the tissues has been performed.

## 11. Postoperative Wound Stress

Postoperative activity can produce excessive tension on the wound during the healing phase. Therefore, it is sometimes necessary to immobilize the wound to prevent suture breakdown and **dehiscence** (breakdown) of the wound. Wound breakdown can occur if the patient coughs or strains postoperatively. Immobilization of the wound can facilitate healing and minimize scar formation.

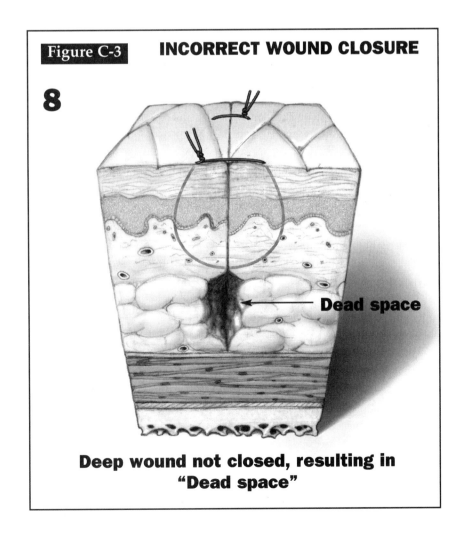

**Figure C-3**   **INCORRECT WOUND CLOSURE**

**8**

← **Dead space**

**Deep wound not closed, resulting in "Dead space"**

# D. Local Anesthetics

## 1. Anesthetics

Local anesthetics are used extensively in surgery. When used in combination with **vasoconstrictive** agents they may reduce surgical blood loss. They can also reduce **perioperative** and **postoperative** pain, reduce nausea and vomiting associated with general anesthetics, reduce **cardiopulmonary** risk, and allow earlier discharge from the hospital. Patients who are good candidates for local anesthetics are people who can cooperate with the surgeon and calmly follow directions. Patients who are **not** good candidates for local anesthetics include children, anxious adults, severely emotionally disturbed patients, and patients with a language barrier. These individuals should probably have surgery done under general anesthesia.

The mechanism of action of local anesthetic agents is to block nerve conduction. This prevents the sensation of pain. Local anesthetics can be used by infiltration (injection) through various sizes (gauges) and lengths of needles **(Table D-1, Figures D-1 and D-2)**. **Table D-2 and D-3** list the common local anesthetic drugs used for infiltration or for topical application.

Table D-1

### CHART OF COMMON NEEDLE SIZES

Gauge refers to diameter, the needle bore. The smaller the number, the bigger the diameter. Therefore, a 16-gauge needle is a larger bore diameter than a 30-gauge needle. The length of the needle ranges from 1/4" to spinal needles of about 3". **See Figures D-1 and D-2.**

Example of the bore diameter of 18-gauge needle
●
Example of the bore diameter of 20-gauge needle
●
Example of the bore diameter of 22-gauge needle
●
Example of the bore diameter of 24-gauge needle
•
Example of the bore diameter of 26-gauge needle
•
Example of the bore diameter of 30-gauge needle
•
*(note: not exact sizes)*

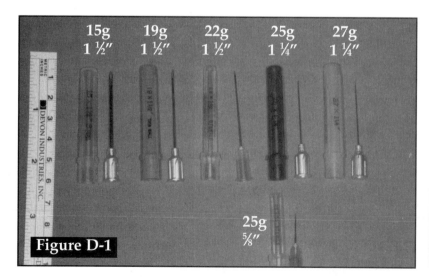

Figure D-1

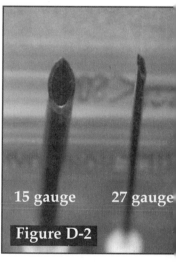

Figure D-2

*Note: various needle lengths and gauge sizes (diameter of bore)*

# D. Local Anesthetics

Table D-2

## Local Anesthetic Drugs for <u>INFILTRATION</u>

| | Maximum dose* without epinephrine by body weight, mg/kg | Onset | Approximate duration | Average adult dose, mg |
|---|---|---|---|---|
| ...docaine (Xylocaine®) | 4.5 mg/kg | Immediate | 2 hours | 500 |
| ...pivacaine (Marcaine®) | 3 mg/kg | 2 to 5 min | 4 hours | 100 |
| ...ocaine (Novocaine®) | 15 mg/kg | 2 to 5 min | 1 hour | 1000 |

...aximum dosage limits must be individualized in each patient. **Epinephrine** is a **vasoconstrictive** agent that ...ows an increased amount of local anesthesia to be injected.

...ample: To calculate the maximum dose of lidocaine the weight of the person must be known.

...r a 70-kg person (154 lb) the maximum dose of lidocaine, with epinephrine is 7 mg/kg (4.5 mg/kg without epi-...phrine). Therefore, 7 mg x 70 kg = 490 mg for a 70-kg person.

... solution = 10 mg/cc**, so 30 cc of 1% lidocaine is safe because 30 cc of 1% lidocaine is 300 mg of lidocaine, ...ich is less than the maximum dose, 490 mg.

**...ARNING:** This table in no way implies that these dosages are safe or absolute maximums. Systemic reactions can be encountered with much ...ller doses, but much larger doses, used judiciously, have been administered without ill effects.

...pted from Moore DC, Bridenbaugh LD, Thompson GE, et al: Factors determining dosages of amide-type local anesthetic drugs. Anesthesiology 1977; ...63-268; in de Jong RH: Local Anesthetics, p 353. St. Louis, Mosby-Year Book, 1994.

...m Brown DL: Regional Anesthesia and Analgesia. p. 140, Section II, Basic Sciences of Regional Anesthetics. W.B. Saunders Co., 1996.

## ** "Kern's Rule"
Percent of drug x 10 = mg of drug per cc

**Example**: *Question*: How many milligrams of lidocaine are there in a 2% lidocaine solution?

*Answer*: A 2% lidocaine solution = 20 mg of lidocaine/cc.

# D. Local Anesthetics

## Table D-3

## Local Anesthetic Drugs for TOPICAL APPLICATION

**For MUCOSA** | **Maximum dose***
| |
Lidocaine (Xylocaine®) | 200 mg (5 cc of a 4% solution)
Cocaine | 200 mg (4 cc of a 5% solution or 2 cc of a 10% solution)
Tetracaine | 100 mg (5 cc of a 2% solution)

**For SKIN --- Local Anesthetic Drugs for Topical Use on Skin**

EMLA Cream  (lidocaine 2.5% plus prilocaine 2.5%)

Apply 1 hour before needle insertion. Duration is 1-2 hours.

Maximum recommended application area is based on body weight:

| Body weight (kg) | Maximum application area, cm$^2$ |
| --- | --- |
| Up to 10 kg | 100 |
| 10 - 20 kg | 600 |
| About 20 kg | 2000 |

***WARNING:**  This table in no way implies that these dosages are safe or absolute maximums.  Systemic reactions can encountered with much smaller doses, but much larger doses, used judiciously, have been administered without ill effects

# D. Local Anesthetics

## 2. Injection technique

There is a method of drawing up the local anesthetic into your syringe. Select a large bore needle (example 18 gauge) to draw the anesthetic solution into your syringe **(Figure D-3)**. First inject about 3 cc of air into the bottle **(Figure D-4)**. Then pull back the plunger of the syringe to draw the anesthetic fluid (solution) into the syringe **(Figure D-5)**. Usually about 5 cc of anesthetic solution is a good start for most procedures.

When inserting local anesthetics it is reasonable to give a **test dose** to make sure no adverse reactions occur. Use the smallest needle size possible to minimize the discomfort. Clean the skin with an alcohol preparation. Penetrate the skin, and advance the needle slowly. Inject and **then** advance so you push the anesthetic into the tissues and **then** advance the needle **(Figure D-6)**. Be sure to discard the needle in a sharps container to prevent accidents. This technique is almost painless when using a 27 g or 30 g (smallest) needle and injecting slowly.

If too much local anesthetic agent is used, toxicity can occur. The signs and symptoms of toxicity must be known by every person who gives these agents. These issues are very important but are beyond the scope of this text.

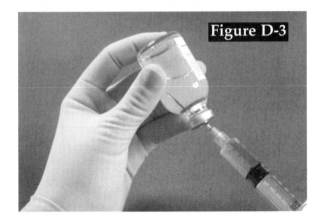

Figure D-3

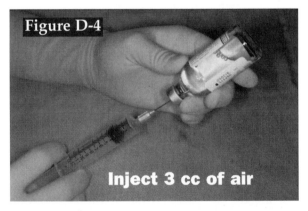

Figure D-4

Inject 3 cc of air

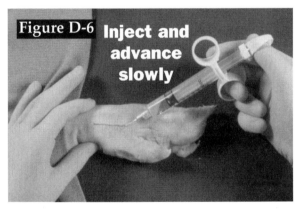

Figure D-6 Inject and advance slowly

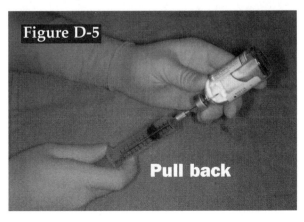

Figure D-5

Pull back

# E. Scrubbing

## 1. *Washing Your Hands*

Prior to scrubbing, always place the surgical scrub suit cap of your choice on your head. All your hair should be covered. Eye protection is required. Be sure to defog your lenses and secure a piece of tape partially over the skin on your nose and partially over your surgical mask to hold the mask in place and minimize fogging of the lenses. Despite different mask styles, they all have a horizontal metal bar that you can tighten over your nose **(Figure E1-2)** to prevent fogging. Now find the scrub sink **(Figure E-3).**

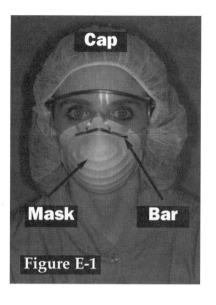

Figure E-1

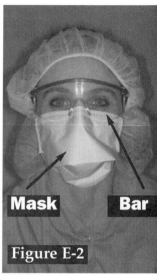

Figure E-2

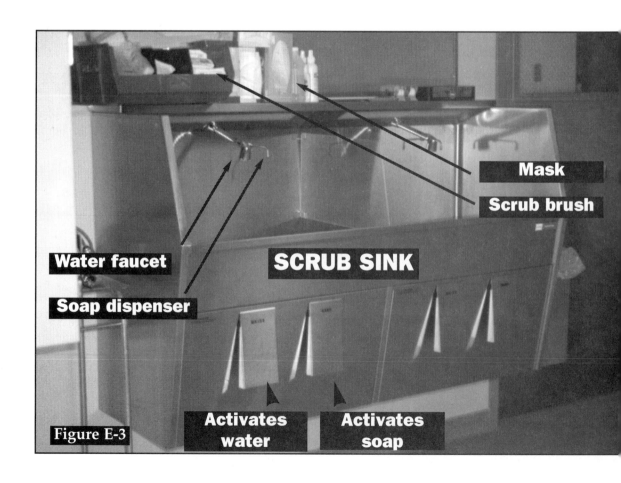

Figure E-3

# E. Scrubbing

The soap, brush and sponge combination are frequently prepackaged. Open the package **(Figures E 4-6)**. The water is turned on by either an automatic switch or a foot or leg switch **(Figure E-7)**. A nail cleaner is typically enclosed in the package. The fingernails are cleaned. Both forearms are wetted up to the elbows, and the foam is formed on the brush **(Figures E-8-11)**.

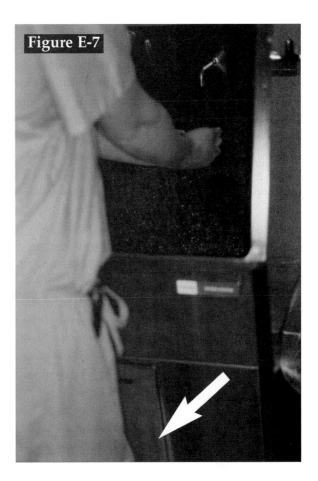

Figure E-7

*Knee activates water flow and turns it off.*

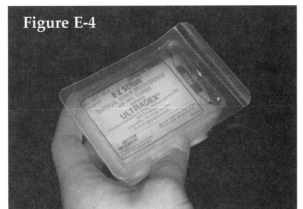

Figure E-4

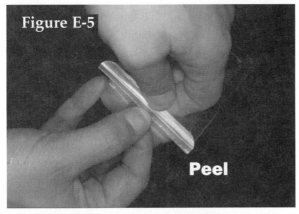

Figure E-5

Peel

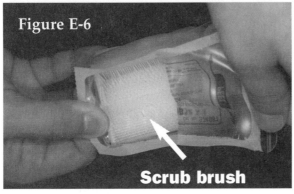

Figure E-6

Scrub brush

# E. Scrubbing

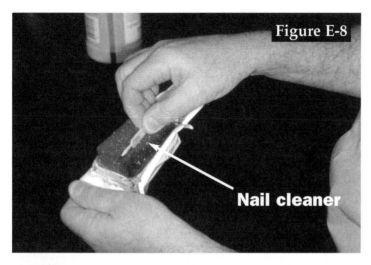

Figure E-8

Nail cleaner

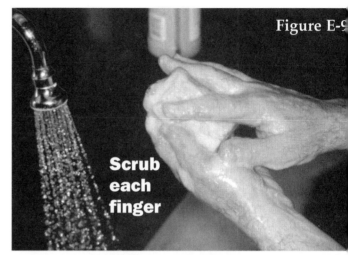

Figure E-9

Scrub
each
finger

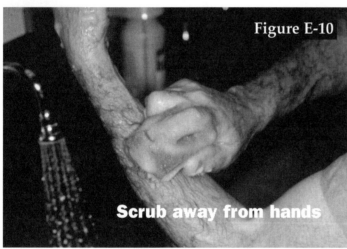

Figure E-10

Scrub away from hands

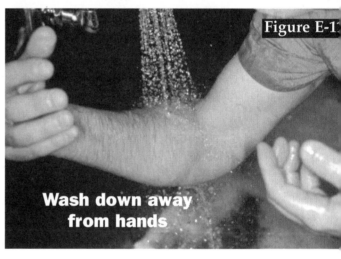

Figure E-11

Wash down away
from hands

After the fingernails are cleansed, the sponge is used to scrub each finger on one hand (**Figure E-9**). The scrub is then carried further up the hands and forearms (**Figure E-10**). The scrub is carried up to the level of the elbow. The other hand is then done in the same fashion with care to clean all sides of the fingers, between the fingers, the hands, wrists, forearms, and up to the elbows. The sponge is discarded, and the hands are first raised, then rinsed.

You can bend over to rinse the arms while holding your hands upright so that the wat runs towards the elbow, **not** back down toward the hand. Why not? The hands are held upright to prevent the soap and water adjacent to the unscrubbed, unsterile elbow region from running back and contaminating the hands (**Figure E-11**).

One arm is then dried from the fingers and hands **toward** the forearm and elbow. The towel is then turned and grasped in the cle area. The same drying procedure is carried out on the opposite arm and hand. Care is taken **NEVER** to dry back from the unsteri elbow region toward the clean hands.

# E. Scrubbing

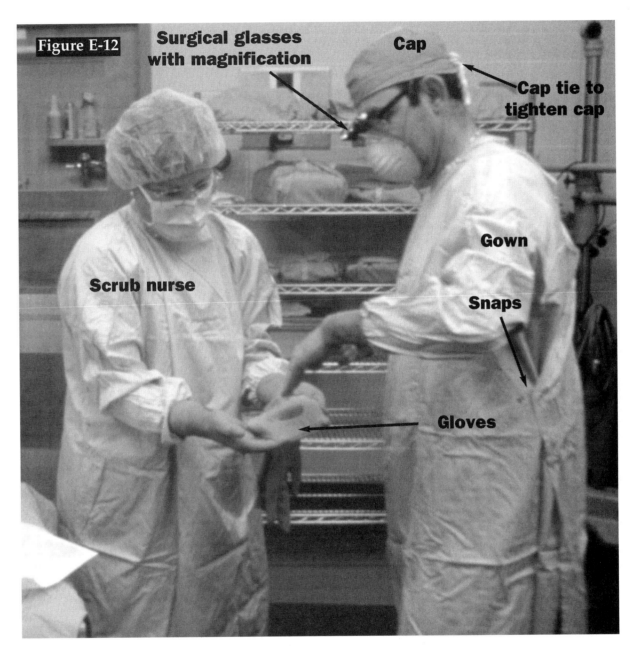

**Figure E-12**

Surgical glasses with magnification

Cap

Cap tie to tighten cap

Gown

Snaps

Scrub nurse

Gloves

## 2. Gowning

The scrub nurse holds up the gown and the surgeon inserts his/her arms. The sterile assistant pulls the gown sleeves so that the surgeon's hands become exposed.

## 3. Gloving

Gloves come in various sizes. The most common sizes range from the smaller 6 1/2 to the larger 8. Try a few sizes to see which is best for you. After the gown is put on, the gloves are held open by the scrub nurse for sterile entry **(Figure E-12)**. Utilizing the first gloved hand, the surgeon can assist the placement of the second glove. A circulating nurse then snaps up the gown for the surgeon. The sterile ties around the gown or snaps can be fixed either by the surgeon or by the scrub nurse to preserve sterility.

# F. Surgical Instruments

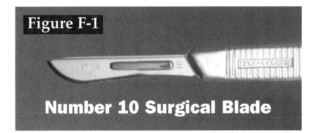
**Figure F-1**

**Number 10 Surgical Blade**

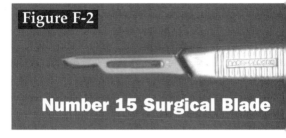
**Figure F-2**

**Number 15 Surgical Blade**

## 1. Scalpel

The scalpel is almost synonymous with the surgeon. It is composed of a scalpel blade and a handle. Scalpels are used to make incisions in the skin or other deeper structures when a fine and precise cut is required. Scalpel blades can also be used to dissect (separate) various types of tissue.

Scalpel blades come in multiple shapes and sizes. The two most common blades are the #10 **(Figure F-1)** and the #15 **(Figure F-2)**.

The Number 10 blade is a large knife blade used for incisions on the scalp and body. The belly of the blade is the cutting edge. The scalpel handle is held like a steak knife **(Figure F-3)**: the index finger guides the blade while the handle is held between the middle finger and thumb in the palm of the hand.

The Number 15 blade is a smaller knife blade. It is typically used for facial surgery. This blade is held like a pencil **(Figure F-4)**. An incision is started by inserting the blade into the skin like a stab. Then the knife handle is rotated backwards so the cutting belly of the blade is held at approximately a 45-degree angle to the skin surface during the incision.

How do you load a scalpel blade onto a scalpel handle? Answer: Grasp the blade with a hemostat clamp near the base of the sharp cutting edge of the blade **(Figure F-5)**. Then advance the blade onto the scalpel handle **(Figure F-5)**. To unload the scalpel blade the blade is again grasped with the hemostat clamp **(Figure F-6)**, then rotate the hemostat clamp to lift the blade and advance (push) forward and remove the blade **(Figure F-6)**.

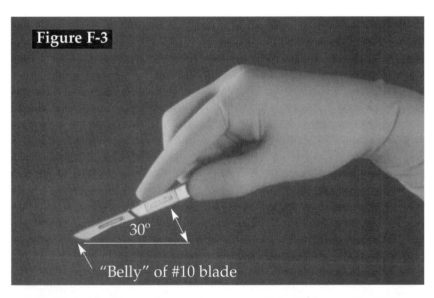
**Figure F-3**

30°

"Belly" of #10 blade

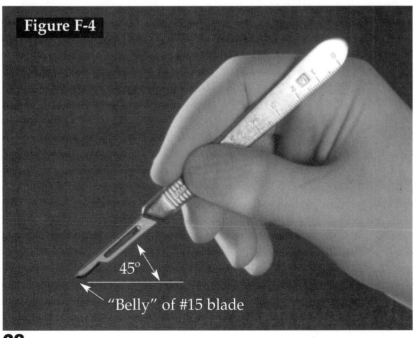
**Figure F-4**

45°

"Belly" of #15 blade

# F. Surgical Instruments

## LOADING THE SCALPEL

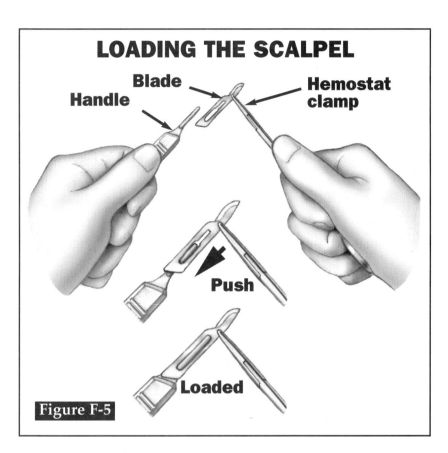

Handle    Blade    Hemostat clamp

Push

Loaded

Figure F-5

## UNLOADING THE SCALPEL

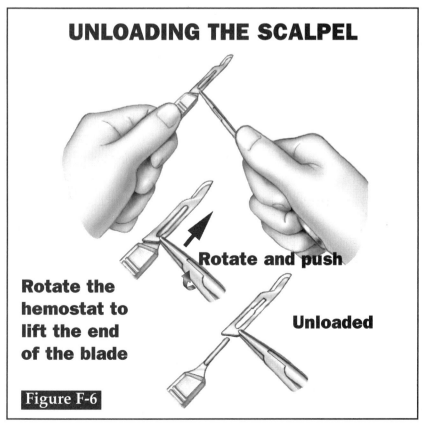

Rotate and push

Rotate the hemostat to lift the end of the blade

Unloaded

Figure F-6

# F. Surgical Instruments

## 2. Tissue Scissors

Tissue scissors (also called dissection scissors or undermining scissors) are used to separate (dissect) the tissues. This elevation or separation of the tissues is called undermining. Many tissue scissors are curved at the cutting edge **(Figures F-7-9)**. If they are curved at the cutting edge, it is best to dissect and undermine with the curved tips **upward** so you can visualize exactly what is being cut. Dissection scissors usually have tips that are either partially blunted or fully blunted to prevent penetration of structures beyond the surgeon's view **(Figures F-8, 9)**. When dissecting with tissue scissors, appropriate tension and countertension on the wound edges are necessary for precise undermining.

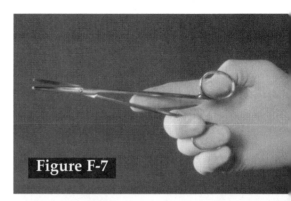

Figure F-7

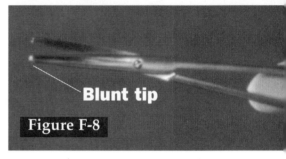

**Blunt tip**

Figure F-8

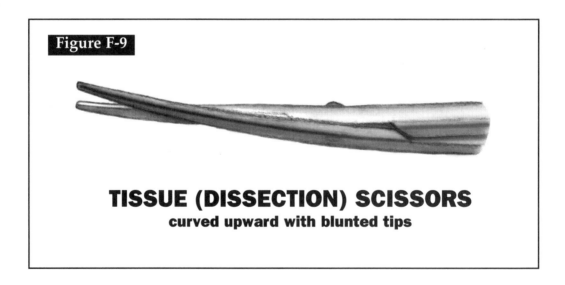

Figure F-9

## TISSUE (DISSECTION) SCISSORS
### curved upward with blunted tips

# F. Surgical Instruments

## 3. Forceps

The forceps is used to grasp, retract, or stabilize tissue. The forceps is gripped between the thumb and middle finger while the index finger is utilized for stabilization **(Figure F-10)**. Various types of forceps are available. They come either with no teeth, single teeth, or multiple teeth on the end of the instrument **(Figure F-11)**. Various tooth sizes are used depending on the size and nature of the tissues to be handled. When grasping tissue, choose a forceps with a tooth size appropriate for the delicacy of the tissue to be handled **(Figure F-11)**. If possible, when operating on skin, use forceps to grasp the dermis (tissue just below the surface) rather than the epidermis (the skin surface itself). This grasping of the dermis helps to prevent marking and injuring the skin at the wound edge with the forceps.

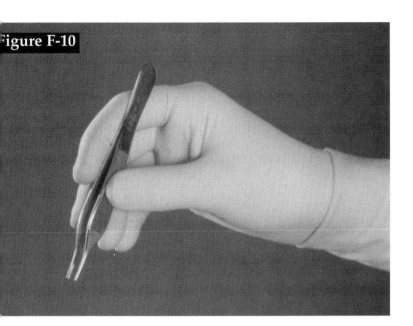

Figure F-10

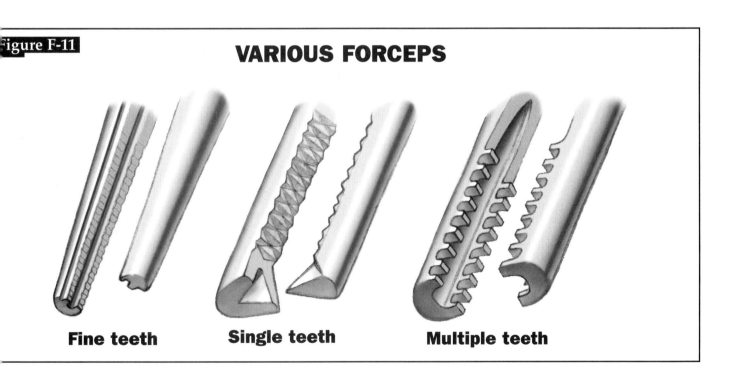

Figure F-11

**VARIOUS FORCEPS**

**Fine teeth**     **Single teeth**     **Multiple teeth**

# F. Surgical Instruments

## 4. Skin Hooks

Skin hooks are used for pulling (also called retracting) tissues **(Figure F-12)**. Retracting allows you to see the deeper tissues, and also puts the tissues on tension, which can help in the surgical dissection with a knife or tissue scissors. Most skin hooks have small, sharp prongs that hook into the dermis. This prevents trauma to the epidermis during wound retraction.

The hooks are placed and retraction is performed by grasping the instrument between the thumb and index finger. The middle finger can stabilize the hook **(Figure F-13)** or can be used to place countertraction on the tissue beyond the skin hook for better visibility and easier dissection.

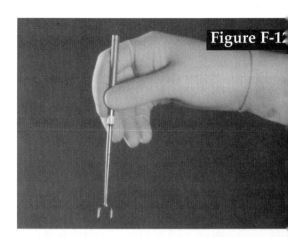

Figure F-12

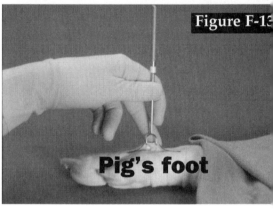

Figure F-13

Pig's foot

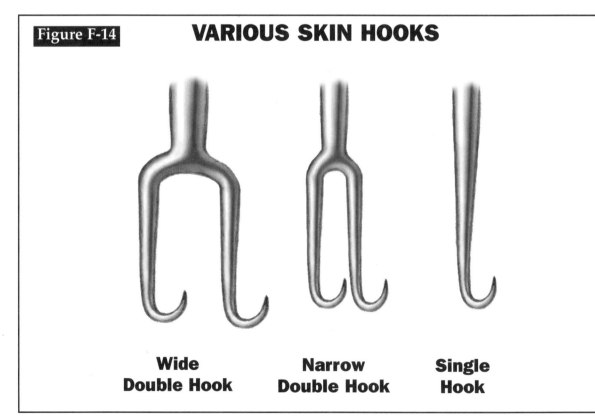

Figure F-14    **VARIOUS SKIN HOOKS**

**Wide Double Hook**    **Narrow Double Hook**    **Single Hook**

# F. Surgical Instruments

## 5. Retractor

The retractor is a blunt instrument used to pull tissues out of the way **(Figure F-15)**. They come in all shapes and sizes and some are even self-retaining.

Pulling the tissue in one direction is called traction. Pulling the tissue in opposite directions is called counter-traction. Both traction and counter-traction can be accomplished with either an instrument or finger (pulling with tension) **(Figure F-16)**.

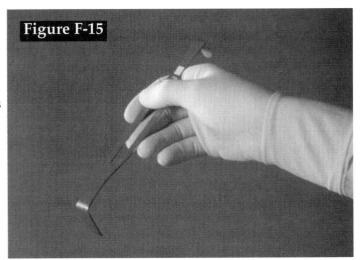

Figure F-15

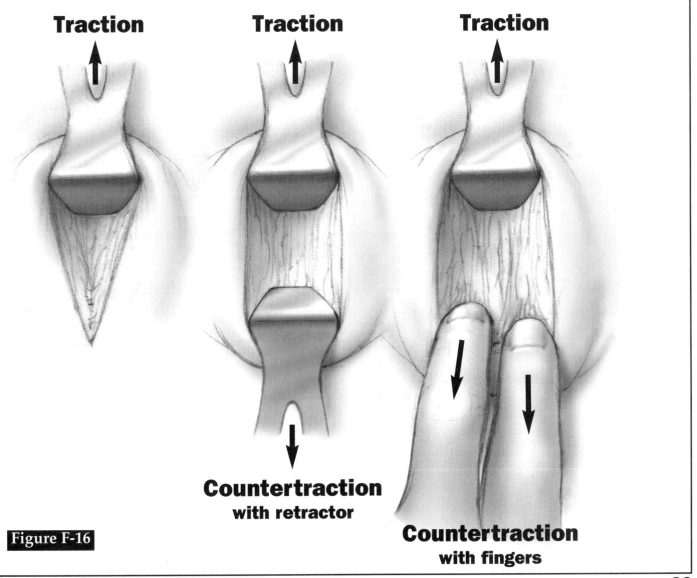

**Traction**

**Traction**

**Traction**

**Countertraction**
**with retractor**

**Countertraction**
**with fingers**

Figure F-16

# F. Surgical Instruments

## 6. Needle Holder (Needle Driver)

The needle holder is the instrument used for placing sutures. Actually, the needle holder, also called a needle driver, holds the needle and pushes or drives the needle with the attached suture through the tissues.

The needle holder is held in the palm with the thumb and fourth finger in the rings (holes) of the handle (Figure F-17). The second finger is utilized to stabilize the direction of the needle holder's end. The third finger is placed against the ring, with the fourth finger used to stabilize the holding of the needle holder.

The needle with the suture attached is usually grasped in the jaws of the needle hold at about two-thirds from the pointed tip o the needle (Figure F-18). This allows stabilization of the needle and helps prevent bending of the needle.

Needle holders may have several varieties jaws (Figure F-19). The first are jaws with teeth. These contain particles such as tungsten carbide for needle stability and prevent rotation or slipping of the needle in the jaw Second are smooth jaws (without teeth). A smooth, fine-jawed needle holder is used with fine needles, and a heavier, wider-jawed needle holder with teeth is selected a heavier needle. The needle holder can al be used to tie and knot sutures. **Do not** use a hemostat as a needle holder. Hemostat jaws are not designed to hold a needle and may **damage** the needle.

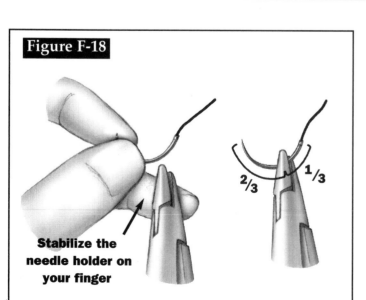

**Figure F-17**

Stabilize the needle holder with index (second) finger

**Figure F-18**

Stabilize the needle holder on your finger

2/3 1/3

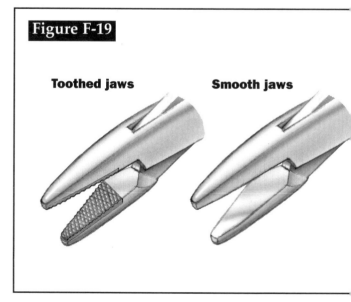

**Figure F-19**

Toothed jaws          Smooth jaws

# F. Surgical Instruments

## 7. Hemostat

The hemostat is a clamp designed to grasp blood vessels prior to cauterization or ligation. The instrument is held much like a needle holder. The hemostat is held in the palm of the hand with the thumb and fourth finger in the rings (holes) of the handle **(Figure F-20)**.

When clamping a blood vessel to stop bleeding you should clamp just the blood vessel and avoid clamping excessive surrounding tissue **(Figure F-21A)**. A blood vessel is clamped with the curved tips of two hemostats **facing** each other **(Figure F-21B)**. The vessel is cut between the two hemostats.

**(Figure F-21C,D)**. Hemostasis is achieved by tying suture around the blood vessel. This tying of suture around a blood vessel is called a vessel ligature.

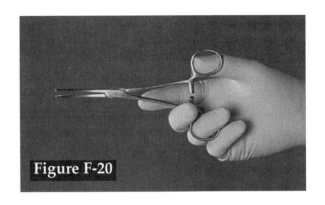

Figure F-20

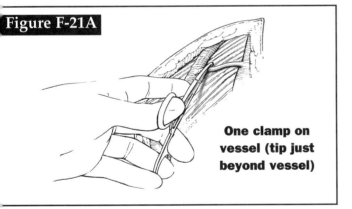

Figure F-21A

One clamp on vessel (tip just beyond vessel)

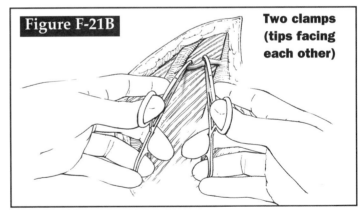

Figure F-21B

Two clamps (tips facing each other)

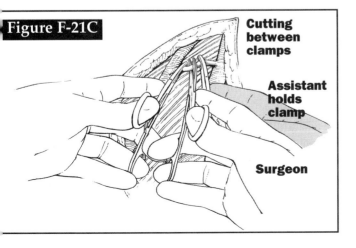

Figure F-21C

Cutting between clamps

Assistant holds clamp

Surgeon

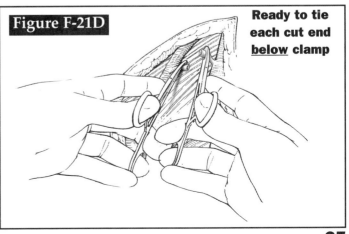

Figure F-21D

Ready to tie each cut end below clamp

# F. Surgical Instruments

## 8. Suction

There are various suction instruments used to remove fluids and blood from the surgical field **(Figures F-22, 23)**. Some suctions are continuous while others are intermittent. Continuous suction does not have a side port and produces a sustained and continuous suction effect **(Figure F-24)**. The intermittent suctions have a side port hole that can be plugged (occluded) which allows the suction effect to occur. When the side port hole is unplugged, the suction is turned off.

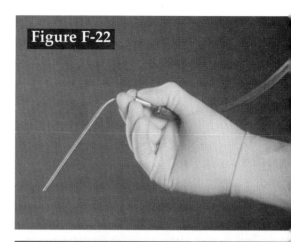

**Figure F-22**

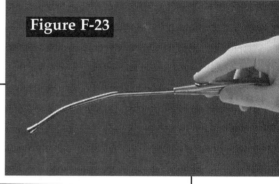

**Figure F-23**

**Figure F-24**

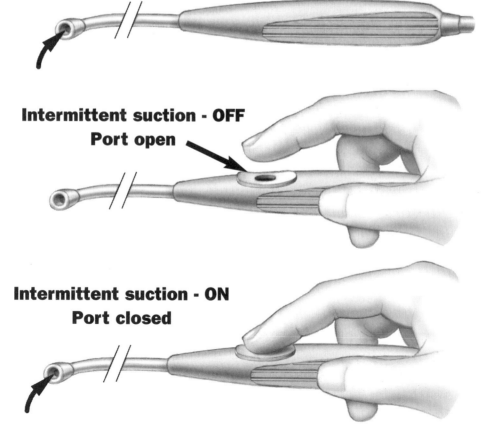

**Continuous suction**
**No port**

**Intermittent suction - OFF**
**Port open**

**Intermittent suction - ON**
**Port closed**

# F. Surgical Instruments

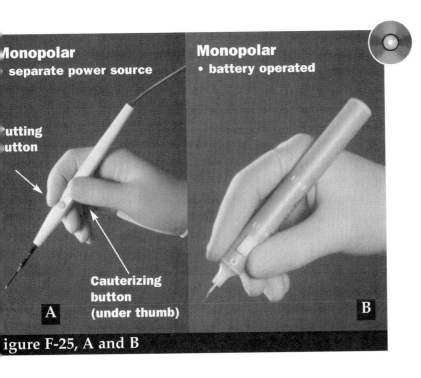

**Monopolar**
• separate power source

Cutting button

Cauterizing button (under thumb)

**A**

**Monopolar**
• battery operated

**B**

Figure F-25, A and B

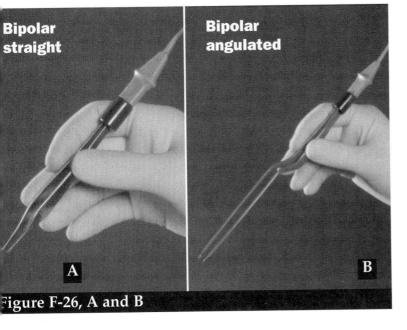

**Bipolar straight**

**A**

**Bipolar angulated**

**B**

Figure F-26, A and B

## 9. Cautery

A cautery is an instrument used to coagulate (cauterize) and cut tissue. Cautery is an electrical current which coagulates the blood vessels to arrest bleeding. There are two types of cautery: monopolar and bipolar. The monopolar cautery generates more heat than the bipolar cautery.

**a. Monopolar cautery** is a cautery with one pole. The current can be used to both cauterize (coagulate) and to cut tissues **(Figure F-25, A)**. There are two types. One is powered by a separate electrical source while the other is battery operated. Both types are disposable **(Figure F-25, A and B)**. Press the button to activate the electric current. Cautery is rarely used to cut skin. Occasionally the cautery will be used to incise and cauterize the deeper tissues for speed and hemostasis.

**b. Bipolar cautery** is a cautery with two poles, one on each side of a forceps-like instrument. Basically there are two types of bipolar cautery. One is straight **(Figure F-26, A)** and the other is angulated **(Figure F-26, B)**. The tissue that is grasped in the forceps of the bipolar cautery is cauterized. Using a bipolar cautery is more precise and results in less transmission of heat to surrounding tissues. A bipolar cautery is usually activated by a foot pedal.

# F. Surgical Instruments

## 10. Suture Scissors

Suture scissors are used to cut suture. You will probably use the suture scissors as the first instrument of initial surgical experience **(Figure F-27)**.

Sutures that are buried are left within the body. These sutures are usually cut on the knot **(Figure F-28)**. Cutting on the knot cuts the tails off the ends of the suture. To accomplish this, you slide the suture scissors down the suture until the knot is felt just under the blades of the suture scissors. Then the scissors are turned slightly and the suture is cut flush on the knot **(Figure F-28)**.

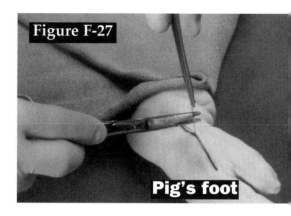

Figure F-27

Pig's foot

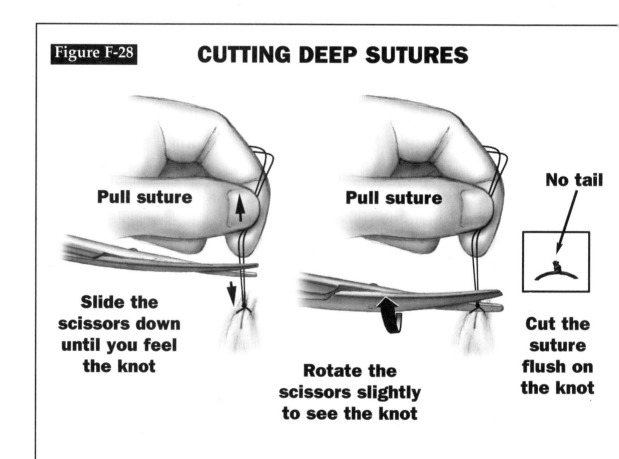

Figure F-28

## CUTTING DEEP SUTURES

**Pull suture**

**Slide the scissors down until you feel the knot**

**Pull suture**

**Rotate the scissors slightly to see the knot**

**No tail**

**Cut the suture flush on the knot**

# F. Surgical Instruments

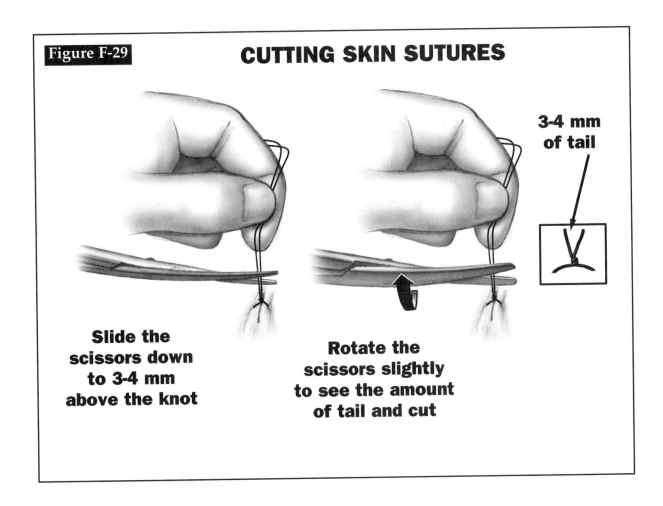

**Figure F-29**

## CUTTING SKIN SUTURES

Slide the
scissors down
to 3-4 mm
above the knot

Rotate the
scissors slightly
to see the amount
of tail and cut

3-4 mm
of tail

When a tail is to be left behind, especially on skin sutures, slide the scissors down the suture to the appropriate tail length, turn, and then cut. This turning of the scissors allows the surgical assistant to visualize the knot and the amount of tail that will be left behind **(Figure F-29)**. This technique ensures the proper length of the tail that is left behind. Usually an appropriate tail length for skin sutures is about three or four millimeters.

Why is a tail left? Leaving three to four millimeters of a suture tail helps prevent loosening, knot slippage, and undoing of the sutures. Grasping the tail with forceps also facilitates suture removal postoperatively. To remove a suture you lift the suture with a forceps, cut with scissors and remove the suture, usually 5 - 14 days later.

# F. Surgical Instruments

### 11. Towel Clip

A towel clip is used to hold surgical drapes and towels together. It is held like a hemostat **(Figure F-30)**. During draping of the patient to prepare the surgical field, drapes are held in place most often with towel clips.

### 12. Staple Gun

The hand-held disposable staple gun is used to apply metal staples to close the skin **(Figure F-31)**. This is especially useful for rapid closure of many incisions. Staples are never used in the face.

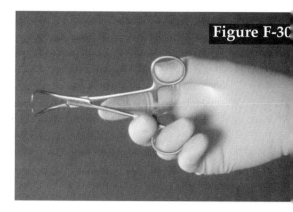

Figure F-30

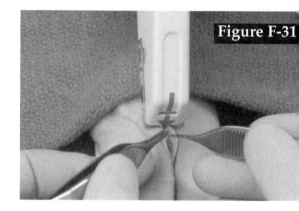

Figure F-31

# Quiz

Fill in the shaded blanks! See page 29, Figure F-5 for the correct answers.

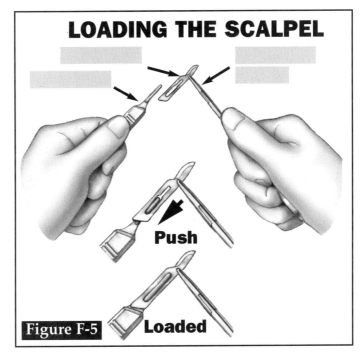

## LOADING THE SCALPEL

Push

Figure F-5   Loaded

Fill in the shaded blanks! See page 39 Figure F-29 for the correct answers.

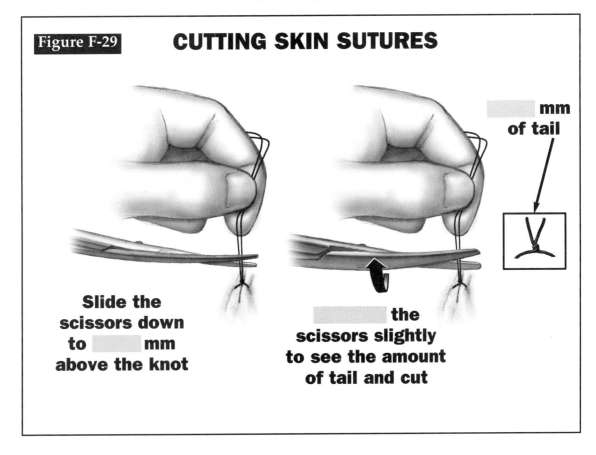

Figure F-29   **CUTTING SKIN SUTURES**

[blank] mm
of tail

Slide the
scissors down
to [blank] mm
above the knot

[blank] the
scissors slightly
to see the amount
of tail and cut

# G. Sutures and Knots

## 1. Introduction

Sutures are materials used to close wounds. Ligatures are materials used to close blood vessels. Sutures and ligatures were used by both the Egyptians and Syrians two thousand years B.C. Suturing was performed even in the time of Hippocrates. Sheep intestines were first mentioned as suture material in the writings of Galen, the Roman physician. The first reports of suturing abdominal wounds appeared in the work of Rhazes, the Arabian surgeon, in approximately 800 A.D. As a surgeon you will hear the term catgut. This is actually a misnomer because it does not refer to cats or guts. Catgut is derived from the Arabic word "kitgut," which refers to the strings of a violin.

After the introduction of anesthetics in the middle of the 19th century and the use of antiseptics by Joseph Lister in 1865, the art and science of surgery progressed rapidly. The development of sutures and suturing techniques paralleled the development of surgery. The early 1950s heralded the introduction of the individually packed, pre-sterilized suture material.

After you complete the deep surgery, you must close the wound. The wound is closed in anatomic layers. The one exception is the wound of the eyelid where the skin and underlying orbicularis oculi muscle layers are extremely thin and can be closed as one layer. Most wounds are closed at each anatomic layer. For example, the incised muscle layers, subcutaneous tissues, and skin are closed separately. The muscle layers and the subcutaneous layers are usually closed with buried, absorbable suture. The skin is usually closed with non-absorbable suture. In high tension wounds, which are wounds that are difficult to bring together, longer lasting absorbable or permanent subcutaneous suture may be required to prevent wound breakdown.

Prior to starting the wound closure, undermining the skin and soft tissues is done to relieve tension at the wound edges. This allows the wound to be approximated and closed without tension. Undermining of one or two centimeters from the wound edge will decrease wound closing tension. The undermining of the soft tissues beyond and below the incision can be done with either a scalpel or scissors. As a young surgeon, you should begin undermining with scissors. This is because you can undermine quickly and safely with the dissection scissors.

What do you need to know about suture materials? Some of the important factors regarding suturing material choice for surgery include diameter, tensile strength, tissue reactivity, the ease of handling the suture material, the facility for tying and maintaining knots, plus the absorption of the sutures by the body.

## 2. Suture Materials

There are a great variety of suture materials, suture sizes, and needle sizes available. Suture materials are divided into absorbable and non-absorbable types. We have tried to simplify the entire topic of suture materials by using the table format to summarize the important points. First, some basic concepts

# G. Sutures and Knots

**ABSORBABLE SUTURES** are dissolved by the body and do not require removal **(Table G-1)**. Absorbable sutures come in polyfilament (braided) and monofilament (unbraided) sutures. Each have various half-lives and strengths. The most common absorbable sutures include gut, polyglycolic acid (Dexon®), polyglactin 9-10 (Vicryl®), polydioxanone (PDS®), and polyglicaprone 25 (Monocryl®). Gut, Dexon®, and Vicryl® are polyfilament sutures, which means that they are braided together for increased strength. While the polyfilament sutures have the advantage of being braided for strength, they have the disadvantage of a "wick effect" that can allow bacterial penetration between the braids of the suture. Monofilament sutures are not braided. Both collagen and surgical gut sutures can be plain or chromic. Chromatizing means that the half-life of the suture will be extended so the suture will stay in place longer. This facilitates wound healing before the sutures lose their tensile strength and fall apart.

Table G-1.
## ABSORBABLE Suture Materials

| ME | MATERIAL | TENSILE STRENGTH | TISSUE$^o$ REACTIVITY | HANDLING$^†$ | KNOT$^\infty$ SECURITY | ABSORPTION |
|---|---|---|---|---|---|---|
| COLLAGEN (plain/chromic) | Beef Tendon | Poor * | +2 | Fair | Poor | 1 to 2 weeks |
| SURGICAL GUT (plain) | Animal Collagen | Poor * | +4 | Fair | Poor | 1 to 2 weeks |
| SURGICAL GUT (chromic) | Animal Collagen | Poor * | +3 | Fair | Fair | 1 to 2 weeks |
| COATED VICRYL ® | Polyglactin 910 Coated Polyglactin 370 and Calcium Sterate | Good ✚ | +1 | Good | Fair | 3 months |
| DEXON "S" ® | Polyglycolic | Good ✚ | +1 | Fair | Good | 3 months |
| PDS ® | Polydioxanone | Good ✚ | +1 | Poor | Poor | 6 months |
| MONOCRYL ® | Polyglicaprone 25 | Fair • | +1 | Good | Good | 3 months |

Poor = absorbed and 0% strength by 3 weeks

Good = 50% strength remains by 3 weeks

Fair = 20% strength remains by 3 weeks

o Tendency to cause inflammation, +1 low, +4 high

† Ease of using suture

∞ Tendency to stay knotted

# G. Sutures and Knots

**NONABSORBABLE SUTURES** are not dissolved by the body and do require removal **(Table G-2)**. In this group, silk is the only braided suture. For this reason, silk may cause microabscesses along the wound edge and is rarely used for epidermal (skin) closure. Nylon and polypropylene are most commonly used for skin closure as well as for buried and long-term "permanent" suture placement. Stainless steel is used to close the sternum of the chest but has few other uses because of its difficult handling properties. Stainless steel staples are excellent for skin closure.

## Table G-2.
## NONABSORBABLE Suture Materials

| NAME | MATERIAL | TISSUE° REACTIVITY | HANDLING† | KNOT ∞ SECURITY | COMMENTS |
|---|---|---|---|---|---|
| 1. SILK | Silk | +4 | Good | Good | |
| 2. ETHILON® | Polyamide (Nylon) | +2 | Fair | Fair | |
| 3. DERMALON® | Polyamide (Nylon) | +2 | Poor | Poor | |
| 4. SURGAMID® | Polyamide (Nylon) | +2 | Poor | Poor | |
| 5. NUROLON® | Polyamide (Nylon) | +2 | Good | Fair | May predispose to infection |
| 6. PROLENE® | Polyolefin (Polypropylene) | +1 | Poor | Poor | Low coefficient of friction |
| 7. MERSILENE® | Polyester | +2 | Good | Good | |
| 8. DACRON® | Polyester | +2 | Good | Good | |
| 9. ETHIBOND® | Polyester (Coated Polybutilate) | +2 | Good | Good | |
| 10. STAINLESS STEEL | Stainless Steel | +1 | Poor* | Good | May kink |

\* Stainless steel staples are an exception since they are well handled with a staple gun.

° Tendency to cause inflammation, +1 low, +4 high

† Ease of using suture

∞ Tendency to stay knotted

# G. Sutures and Knots

Conventional suture package and opening technique to expose inner package with needle and suture are shown (Figures G 1-4).

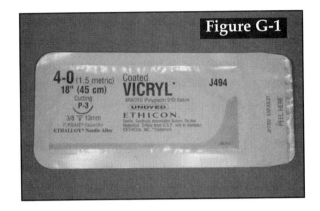

Figure G-1

Some generalizations can be made regarding the best suture choice for the skin closure of a particular body location. **Table G-4** shows suture selection typical for each site. You should always consider using ABSORBABLE sutures in children or the non-compliant adult. Rarely, high tension cutaneous (skin) wounds are closed with 0 or 2-0 sutures. These may be utilized as bolster sutures to help relieve tension on large abdominal wounds.

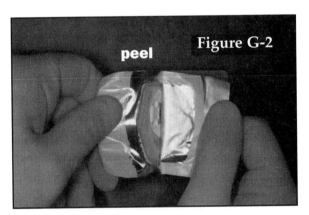

Figure G-2

## Table G-3

The lower the suture size number, the larger (thicker) the diameter and the higher (greater, stronger) the tensile strength.

The higher the suture size number, the smaller (thinner) the diameter and the lower (less, weaker) the tensile strength.

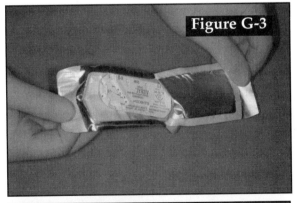

Figure G-3

| Suture Size | Suture Diameter | Tensile Strength |
|---|---|---|
| 1-0 | Larger (thicker) | High (greater, stronger) |
| 2-00 | | |
| 3-000 | | |
| 4-0000 | | |
| 5-00000 | | |
| 6-000000 | | |
| 7-0000000 | | |
| 8-00000000 | | |
| 9-000000000 | | |
| 10-0000000000 | | |
| 11-00000000000 | Smaller (thinner) | Lower (less, weaker) |

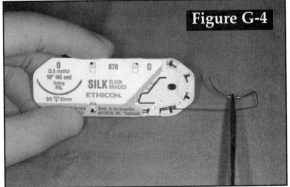

Figure G-4

# G. Sutures and Knots

The size of the suture material is related to the diameter of the suture. This is related to the number of 0s. The lower the suture size number, the larger (thicker) the diameter and the higher (greater, stronger) the tensile strength **(Figure G-3)**. So, a 2-0 or 00 is a much larger diameter suture than a 6-0 or 000000. It should be clear that 2-0 and 00 are alternate ways of saying the same thing. The 2-0 suture has more tensile strength than a 6-0 suture. You should select the smallest diameter suture that can adequately hold the tissue edges together. This will reduce the tissue damage caused by the suture, and the resulting scar will be minimized **(Table G-3)**.

## Table G-4.
## Typical Suture Choices (Suture Size and Suture Material)

| SITE | DEEP LAYERS (SUTURE SIZE) | SUTURE MATERIALS | SKIN LAYERS (SUTURE SIZE) | SUTURE MATERIALS |
|---|---|---|---|---|
| **SCALP** | 2-0 to 4-0 | Absorbable | 4-0 to 5-0 | Nylon, polypropylene, or staples |
| **EYELID** | 5-0 to 7-0 | " | 6-0 to 7-0 | Nylon, polypropylene, plain gut |
| **FACE** | 3-0 to 5-0 | " | 5-0 to 6-0 | Nylon, polypropylene, plain gut |
| **NECK** | 2-0 to 4-0 | " | 4-0 to 5-0 | Nylon, polypropylene, plain gut, or staples |
| **TRUNK** | 2-0 to 3-0 | " | 2-0 to 4-0 | Nylon, polypropylene, or staples |
| **LIMBS** | 2-0 to 4-0 | " | 3-0 to 5-0 | Nylon, polypropylene, or staples |
| **HANDS AND FEET** | 3-0 to 5-0 | " | 4-0 to 5-0 | Nylon, polypropylene, or staples |
| **SOLES OF FEET** | 2-0 to 4-0 | " | 2-0 to 4-0 | Nylon, polypropylene, or staples |

# G. Sutures and Knots

### 3. Needle Types

Common needles used in surgery are (1) tapered and (2) cutting **(Figure G-5)**. The tapered needle has a pointed end, but the rest of the needle itself is a smooth, rounded tube with no cutting edges **(Figure G-5)**. This type of needle is used to minimize trauma to the tissues. It is commonly used in general surgery for closure of mucosal incisions, like those in the stomach or small intestine.

The cutting needle has a sharp end and sharp edges **(Figure G-5)**. Therefore, the entire needle acts as a cutting instrument. The cutting needle is commonly used for subcutaneous, intradermal, and cutaneous (skin) closure. Because of the sharp point and sharp edges, this needle is more amenable to cutting through tougher tissues.

The needles themselves come in various shapes and sizes depending upon their use. Most needles are curved, although straight needles are available for a variety of applications **(Figure G-6)**.

It is important to know how to read the suture package labels. This basic information is found in **Figures G-7-9**.

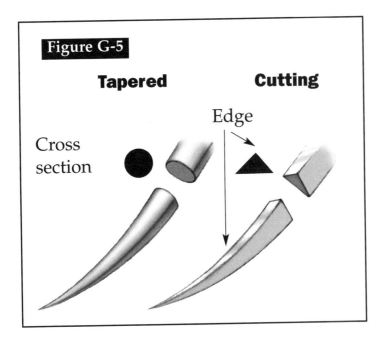

Figure G-5

Tapered

Cutting

Edge

Cross section

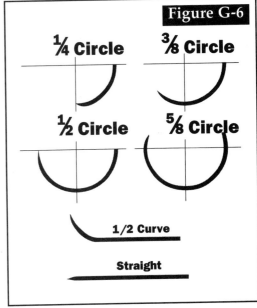

Figure G-6

¼ Circle

⅜ Circle

½ Circle

⅝ Circle

1/2 Curve

Straight

# G. Sutures and Knots

### Figure G-7

## Peelable Foil Pack
Synthetic absorbables only

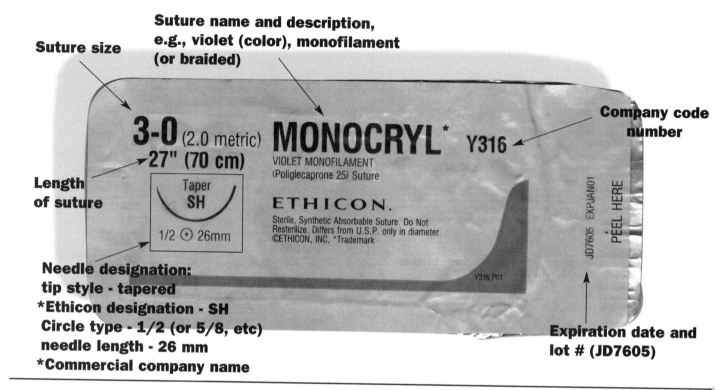

**Suture size**

**Suture name and description, e.g., violet (color), monofilament (or braided)**

**Company code number**

**Length of suture**

**Needle designation:**
tip style - tapered
*Ethicon designation - SH
Circle type - 1/2 (or 5/8, etc)
needle length - 26 mm
*Commercial company name

**Expiration date and lot # (JD7605)**

3-0 (2.0 metric)
27" (70 cm)
Taper SH
1/2 ⊙ 26mm

MONOCRYL* Y316
VIOLET MONOFILAMENT
(Poliglecaprone 25) Suture

ETHICON.
Sterile, Synthetic Absorbable Suture. Do Not Resterilize. Differs from U.S.P. only in diameter.
©ETHICON, INC. *Trademark

JD7605 EXPJAN01   PEEL HERE

Y316.P01

### Figure G-8

## Internal Package
Read the same way

(called "relay package")

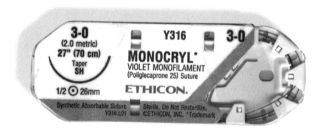

3-0 (2.0 metric)
27" (70 cm)
Taper SH
1/2 ⊙ 26mm

Y316   3-0

MONOCRYL*
VIOLET MONOFILAMENT
(Poliglecaprone 25) Suture

ETHICON.

Synthetic Absorbable Suture   Sterile, Do Not Resterilize.
Y316.L01   ©ETHICON, INC. *Trademark

### Figure G-9

## Conventional Package
Read the same way

**Designates double armed**

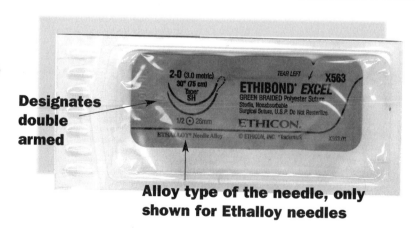

2-0 (3.0 metric)
30" (75 cm)
Taper SH
1/2 ⊙ 26mm

TEAR LEFT   X563

ETHIBOND* EXCEL
GREEN BRAIDED Polyester Suture
Sterile, Nonabsorbable
Surgical Suture, U.S.P. Do Not Resterilize.

ETHICON.
ETHALLOY* Needle Alloy   © ETHICON, INC. *Trademark   X563.01

**Alloy type of the needle, only shown for Ethalloy needles**

48

# G. Sutures and Knots

## 4. Knot Tying

So now you are ready to tie surgical knots. Try to remember back to first learning to tie your shoes as a toddler! At times the skill will come slowly. But once mastered, surgical knot tying will never be forgotten. Please liberally reference the CD-ROM portion of this course during this section. The combination of both still photos and animation should help in acquiring these skills.

**a. Two-Hand Tie**
The two-hand tie is the first type of tie that should be learned. Why? Because it is the most useful. This tie gives the best knot security, especially when compared with the one-hand tie. You must master the two-hand tie early because tying will be one of the first tasks you will be asked to perform as an assistant in surgery. The hand position varies depending upon whether you are a right-handed or left-handed surgeon. The most common types of two-hand ties are the surgeon's knot and the square knot. The knot is considered completed after 3 to 6 throws, depending on the material used and on the surgeon's preference. For instance, silk suture holds a knot well with 3 to 4 throws, while Prolene® suture is only secure after 5 to 7 throws. The CD-ROM module on this subject will be very useful for learning the actual techniques of knot tying; however, we will go through the steps of learning the two-hand tie with illustrations and a piece of string. You can use an armchair and string to learn these knots **(Figure G-10)**. **Figures G-11, G-12 and G-13 (all)** show how to make a square knot.

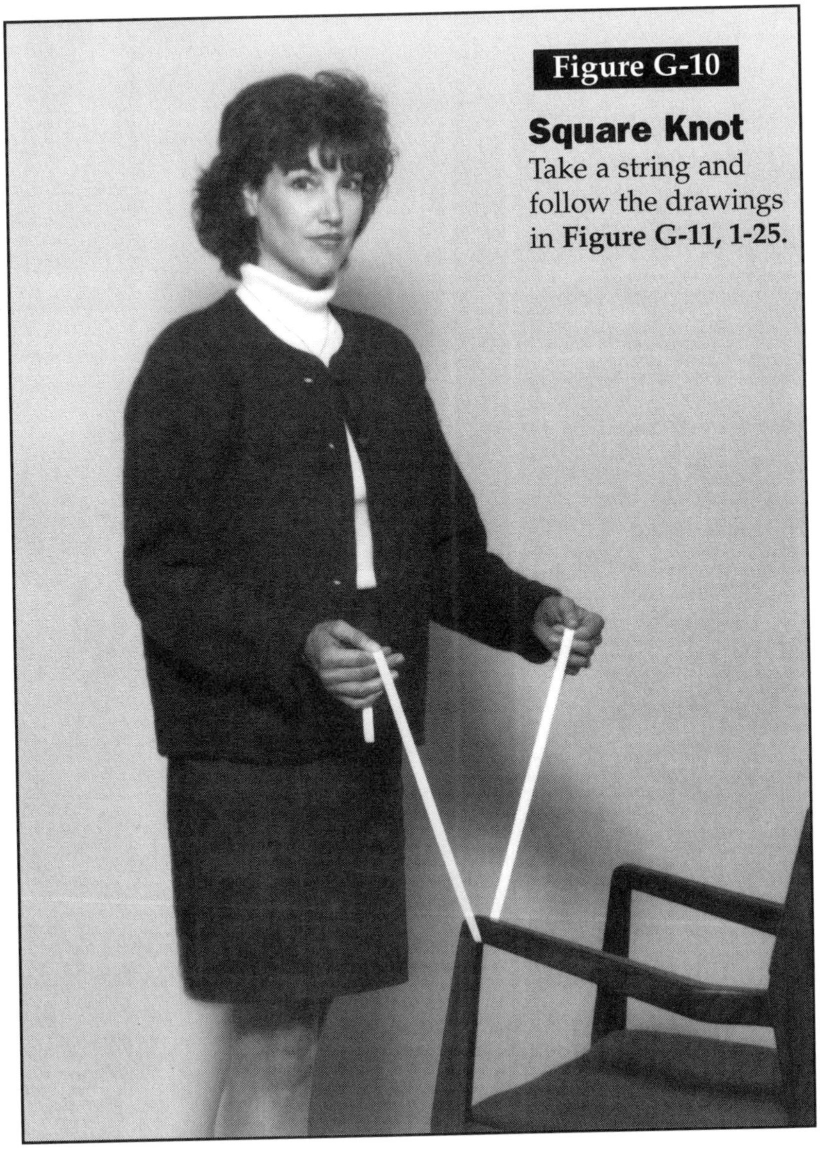

### Figure G-10

**Square Knot**
Take a string and follow the drawings in **Figure G-11, 1-25.**

# G. Sutures and Knots

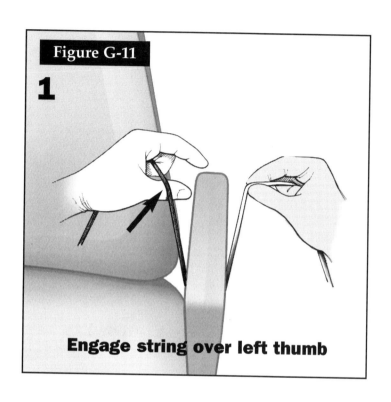

**Figure G-11**

**1**

**Engage string over left thumb**

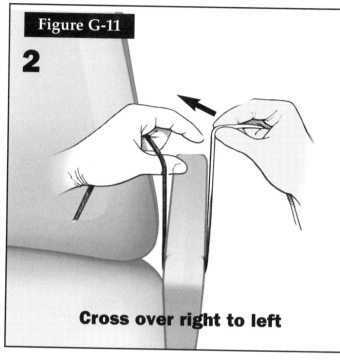

**Figure G-11**

**2**

**Cross over right to left**

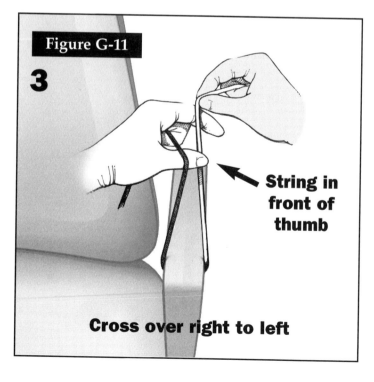

**Figure G-11**

**3**

**String in front of thumb**

**Cross over right to left**

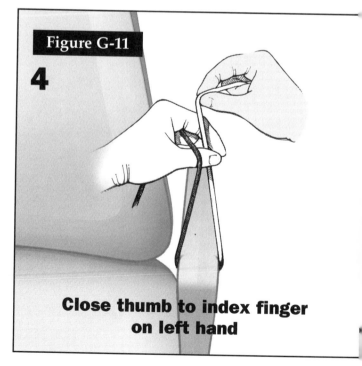

**Figure G-11**

**4**

**Close thumb to index finger on left hand**

50

# G. Sutures and Knots

Figure G-11

**5**

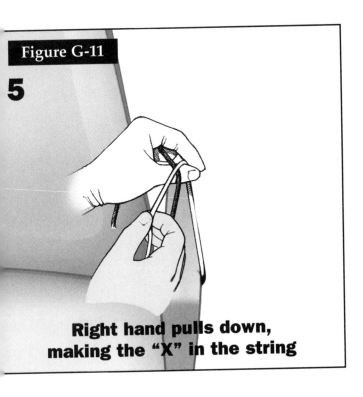

**Right hand pulls down, making the "X" in the string**

Figure G-11

**6**

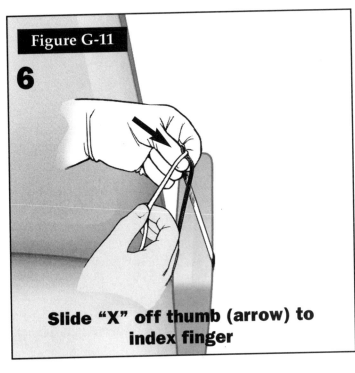

**Slide "X" off thumb (arrow) to index finger**

Figure G-11

**7**

↑ Lift

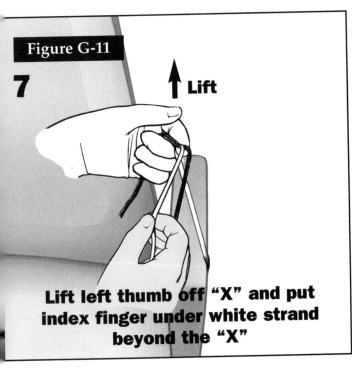

**Lift left thumb off "X" and put index finger under white strand beyond the "X"**

Figure G-11

**8**

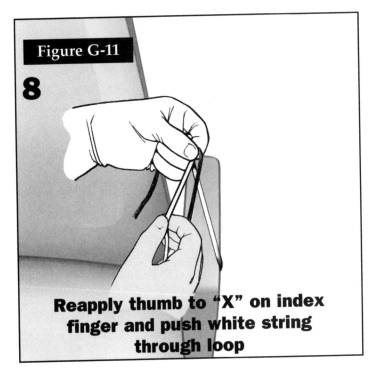

**Reapply thumb to "X" on index finger and push white string through loop**

# *G. Sutures and Knots*

Figure G-11

**9**

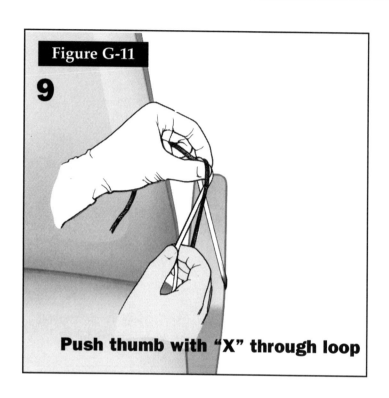

**Push thumb with "X" through loop**

Figure G-11

**10**

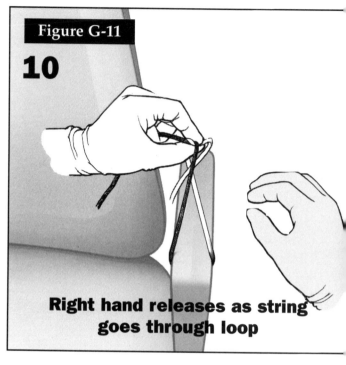

**Right hand releases as string goes through loop**

Figure G-11

**11**

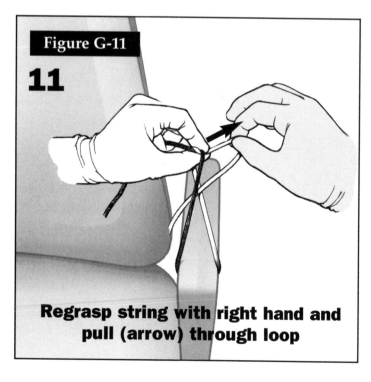

**Regrasp string with right hand and pull (arrow) through loop**

Figure G-11

**12**

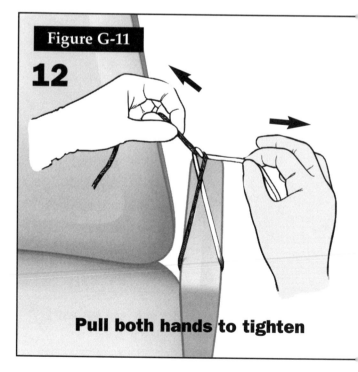

**Pull both hands to tighten**

# G. Sutures and Knots

**Figure G-11**

**13**

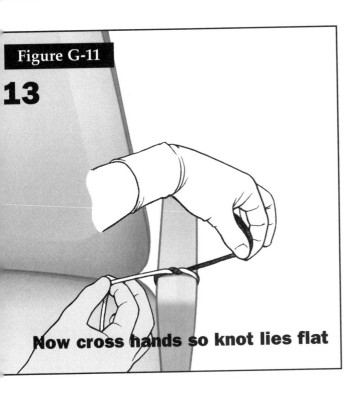

Now cross hands so knot lies flat

**Figure G-11**

**14**

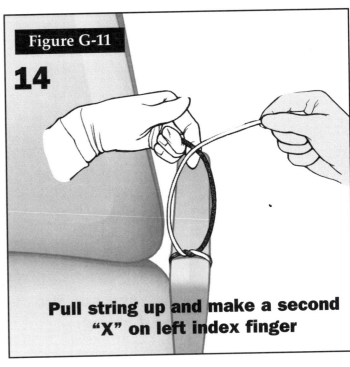

Pull string up and make a second "X" on left index finger

**Figure G-11**

**15**

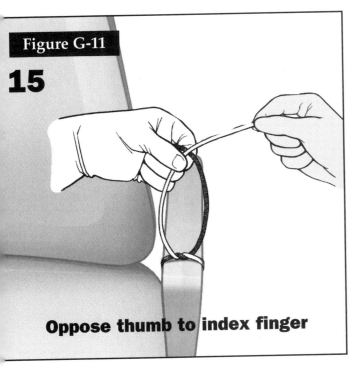

Oppose thumb to index finger

**Figure G-11**

**16**

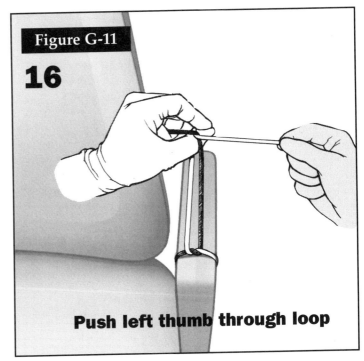

Push left thumb through loop

# G. Sutures and Knots

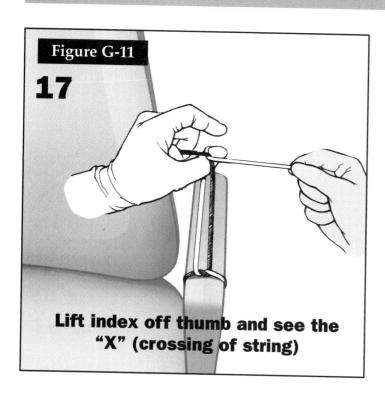

**Figure G-11**

**17**

**Lift index off thumb and see the "X" (crossing of string)**

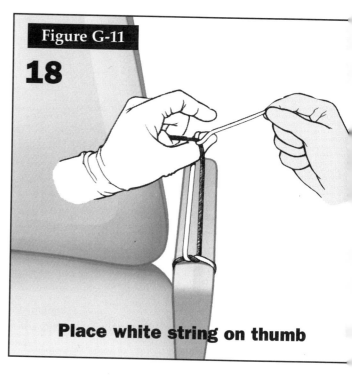

**Figure G-11**

**18**

**Place white string on thumb**

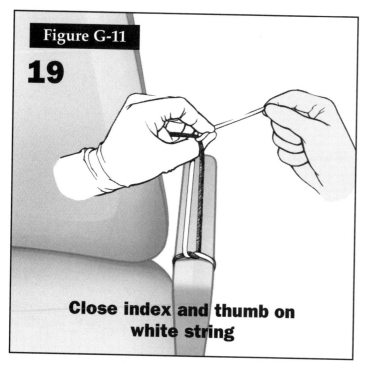

**Figure G-11**

**19**

**Close index and thumb on white string**

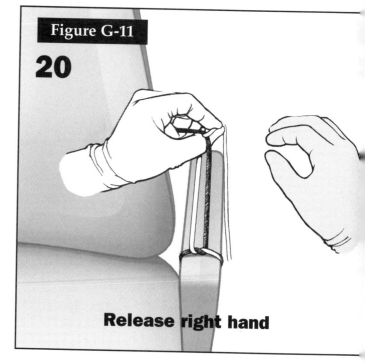

**Figure G-11**

**20**

**Release right hand**

# *G. Sutures and Knots*

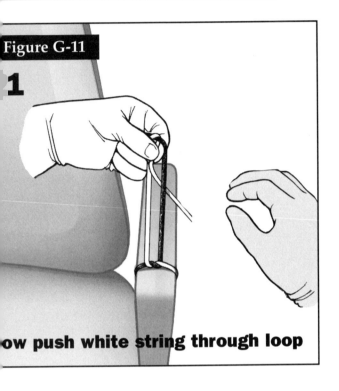

Figure G-11

**1**

ow push white string through loop

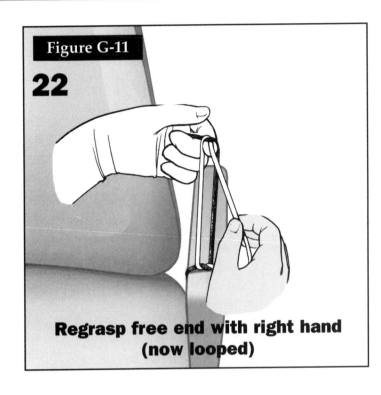

Figure G-11

**22**

**Regrasp free end with right hand (now looped)**

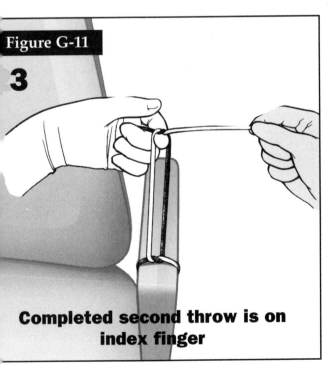

Figure G-11

**3**

**Completed second throw is on index finger**

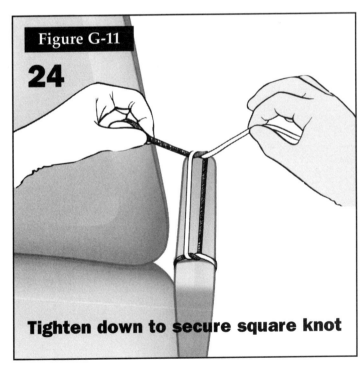

Figure G-11

**24**

**Tighten down to secure square knot**

55

# G. Sutures and Knots

## TWO-HAND TIE — SQUARE KNOT

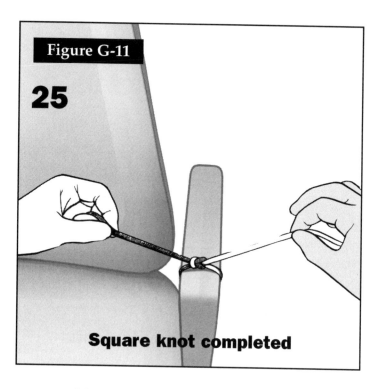

**Figure G-11**

**25**

**Square knot completed**

Most often 4 to 6 throws are placed before a surgeon considers a knot completed. This is to ensure the security of the knot.

**Comparison Between Square Knot and Surgeon's Knot**

The square knot has one loop in the first throw, while the the surgeon's knot has two loops **(Figure G-12:1,2)**. After the first throw is completed the rest of the tie is the same in both knots. Subsequent throws are always opposite the previous throw to improve the security of the tie. When practicing knot tying, do as many throws as the string allows to make the hand motions second nature. The surgeon's knot is useful because the first throw with the two loops **(Figure G-12: 2)** tends to stay in place better than the square knot with its one loop prior to placement of the second throw. **Figure G-12: 3,4** shows the square knot and surgeon's knot secure.

# G. Sutures and Knots

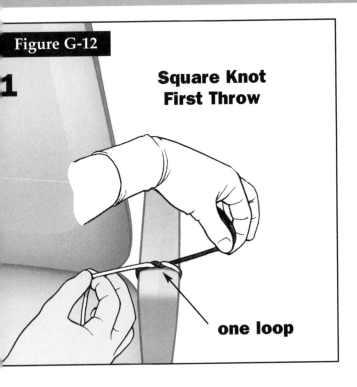

**Figure G-12**

**1**

**Square Knot First Throw**

**one loop**

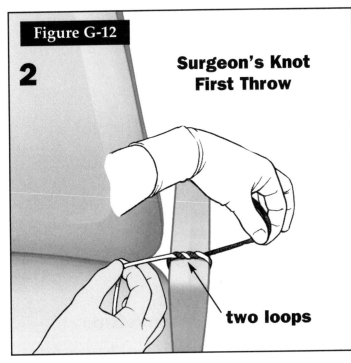

**Figure G-12**

**2**

**Surgeon's Knot First Throw**

**two loops**

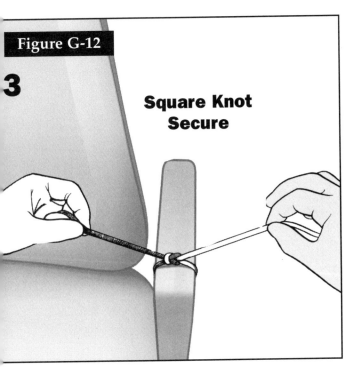

**Figure G-12**

**3**

**Square Knot Secure**

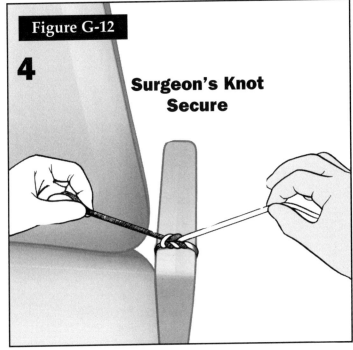

**Figure G-12**

**4**

**Surgeon's Knot Secure**

# G. Sutures and Knots

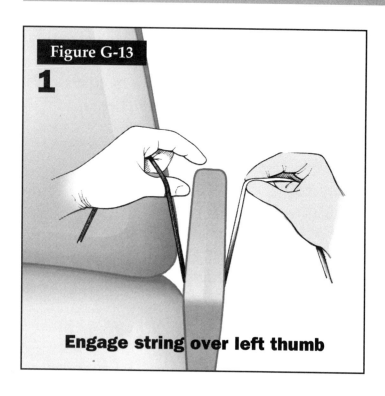

**Figure G-13**

**1**

**Engage string over left thumb**

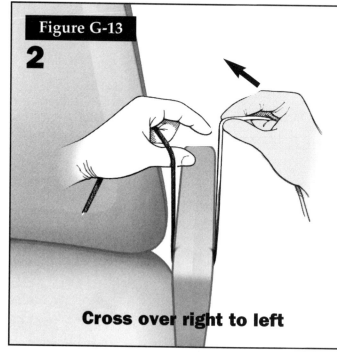

**Figure G-13**

**2**

**Cross over right to left**

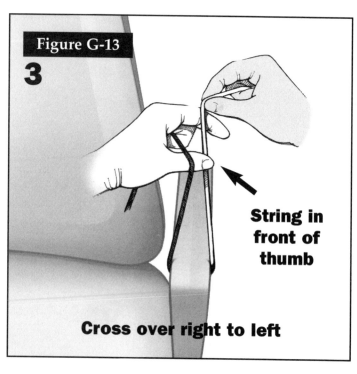

**Figure G-13**

**3**

**String in front of thumb**

**Cross over right to left**

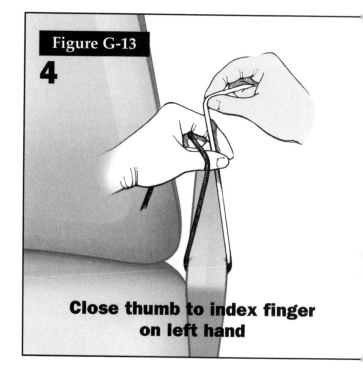

**Figure G-13**

**4**

**Close thumb to index finger on left hand**

# G. Sutures and Knots

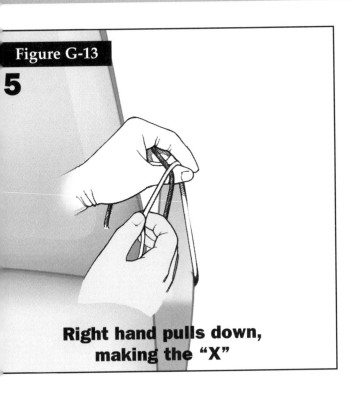

**Figure G-13**

**5**

**Right hand pulls down, making the "X"**

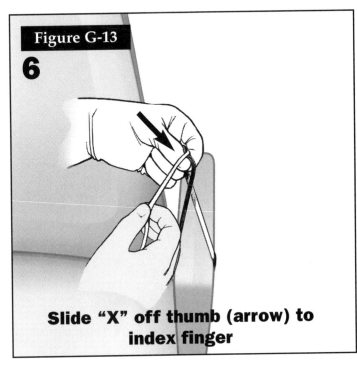

**Figure G-13**

**6**

**Slide "X" off thumb (arrow) to index finger**

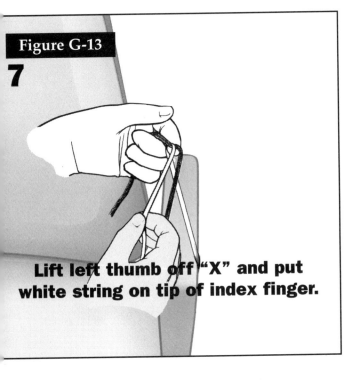

**Figure G-13**

**7**

**Lift left thumb off "X" and put white string on tip of index finger.**

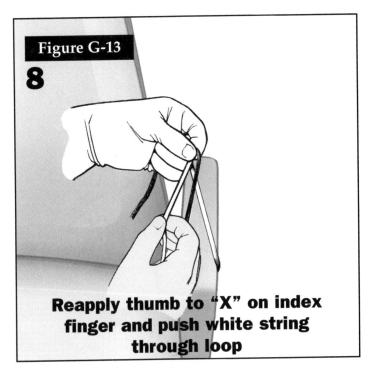

**Figure G-13**

**8**

**Reapply thumb to "X" on index finger and push white string through loop**

# G. Sutures and Knots

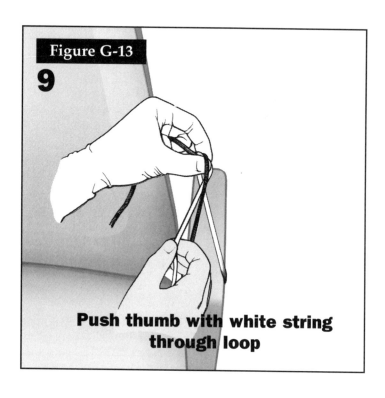

Figure G-13
**9**

**Push thumb with white string through loop**

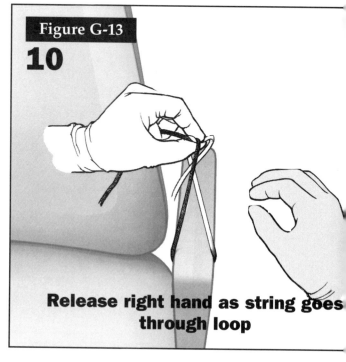

Figure G-13
**10**

**Release right hand as string goes through loop**

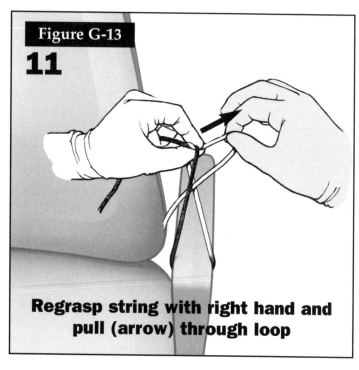

Figure G-13
**11**

**Regrasp string with right hand and pull (arrow) through loop**

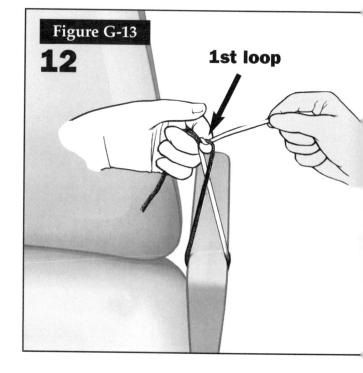

Figure G-13
**12**

1st loop

# G. Sutures and Knots

**Figure G-13**

**13**

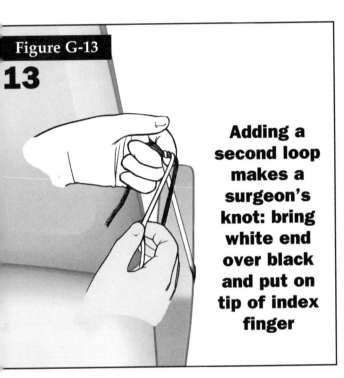

Adding a second loop makes a surgeon's knot: bring white end over black and put on tip of index finger

**Figure G-13**

**14**

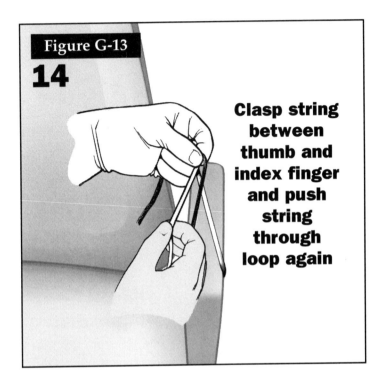

Clasp string between thumb and index finger and push string through loop again

**Figure G-13**

**15**

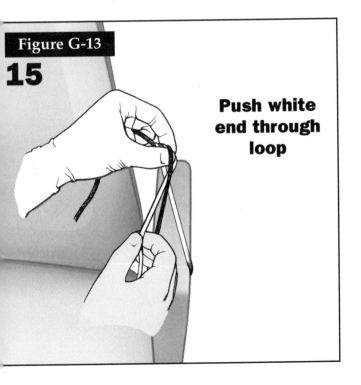

Push white end through loop

**Figure G-13**

**16**

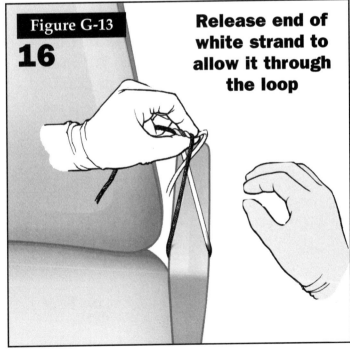

Release end of white strand to allow it through the loop

# G. Sutures and Knots

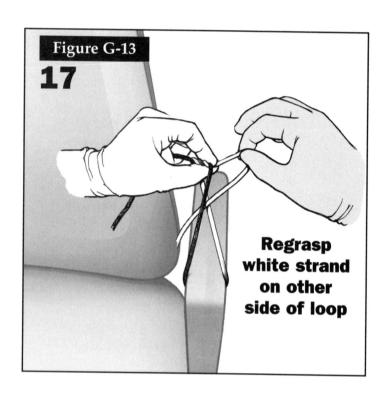

**Figure G-13**
**17**

Regrasp
white strand
on other
side of loop

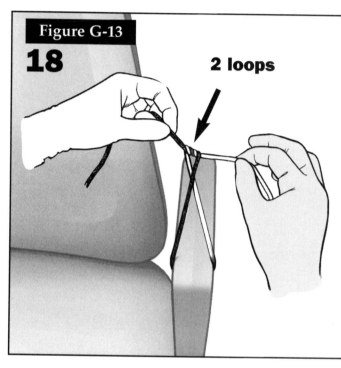

**Figure G-13**
**18**

2 loops

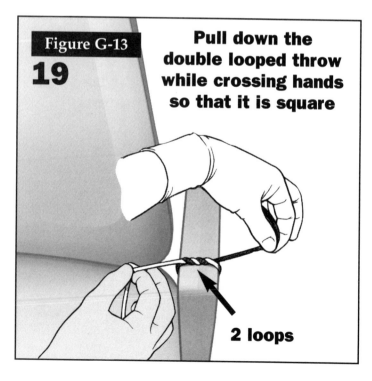

**Figure G-13**
**19**

Pull down the
double looped throw
while crossing hands
so that it is square

2 loops

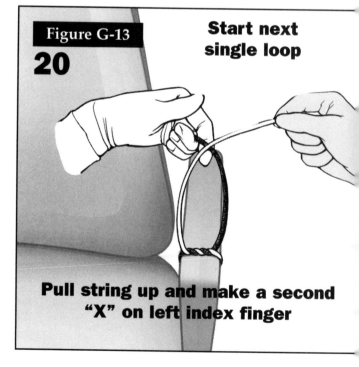

**Figure G-13**
**20**

Start next
single loop

Pull string up and make a second
"X" on left index finger

# G. Sutures and Knots

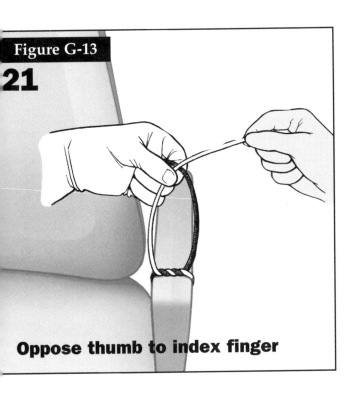

**Figure G-13**
**21**

Oppose thumb to index finger

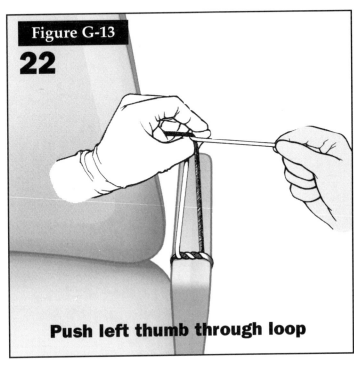

**Figure G-13**
**22**

Push left thumb through loop

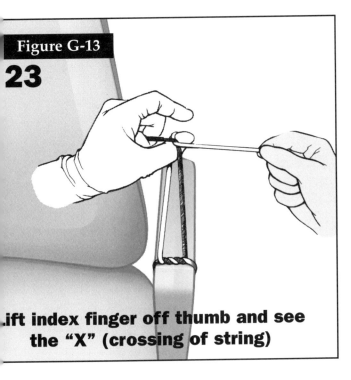

**Figure G-13**
**23**

.ift index finger off thumb and see the "X" (crossing of string)

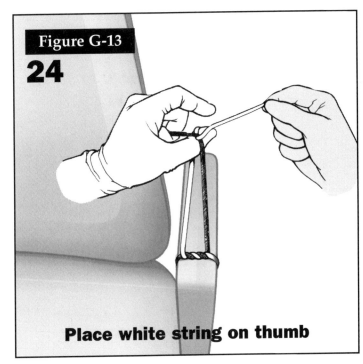

**Figure G-13**
**24**

Place white string on thumb

# G. Sutures and Knots

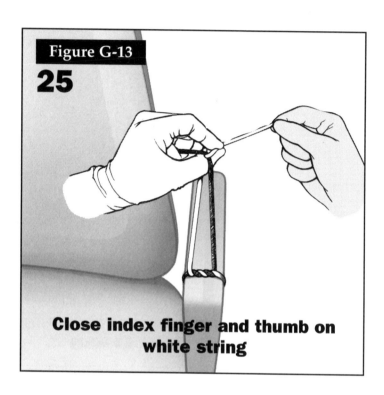

**Figure G-13**

**25**

**Close index finger and thumb on white string**

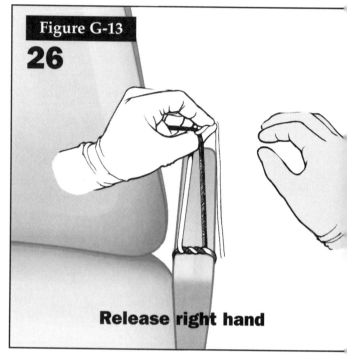

**Figure G-13**

**26**

**Release right hand**

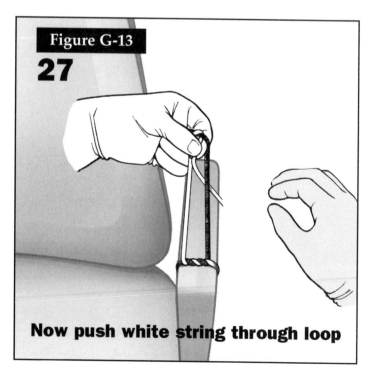

**Figure G-13**

**27**

**Now push white string through loop**

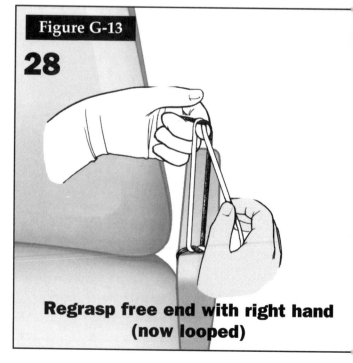

**Figure G-13**

**28**

**Regrasp free end with right hand (now looped)**

# G. Sutures and Knots

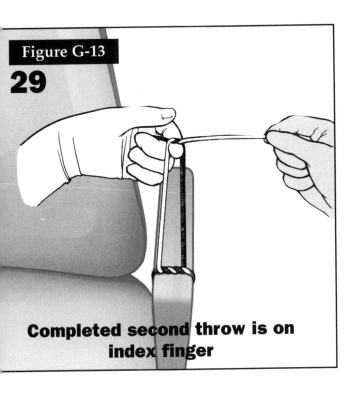

**Figure G-13**
**29**

Completed second throw is on index finger

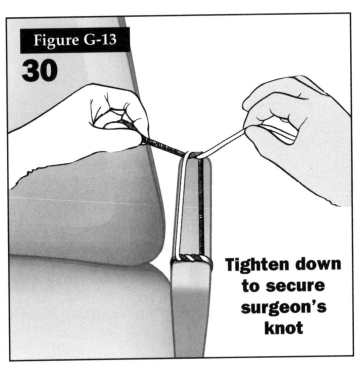

**Figure G-13**
**30**

Tighten down to secure surgeon's knot

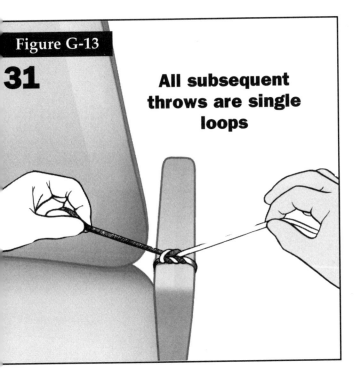

**Figure G-13**
**31**

All subsequent throws are single loops

# G. Sutures and Knots

### b. Instrument Tie

The instrument tie is extremely useful and has a variety of applications, especially in facial surgery. Surgeon's knots and square knots are also used with the instrument tie. In this tie, the needle holder is kept in one hand after passing the needle through the tissue. The suture is then wrapped around the end of the needle holder to make a loop. The short, free end of suture is then grasped in the jaws of the needle holder and pulled through the loop to complete the knot. You can practice the instrument tie by using a silk suture (2-0), a needle holder (driver), and a towel **(Figure G-14: 1-20)**. Two-hand ties can also be practiced with this suture. **IT IS CRITICAL THAT YOU MASTER BOTH OF THESE TYING TECHNIQUES.**

## INSTRUMENT TIE

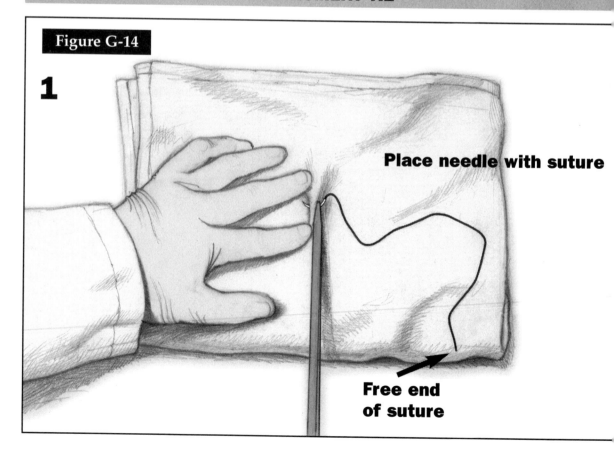

Figure G-14

1

Place needle with suture

Free end of suture

# G. Sutures and Knots

**Figure G-14**

**2**

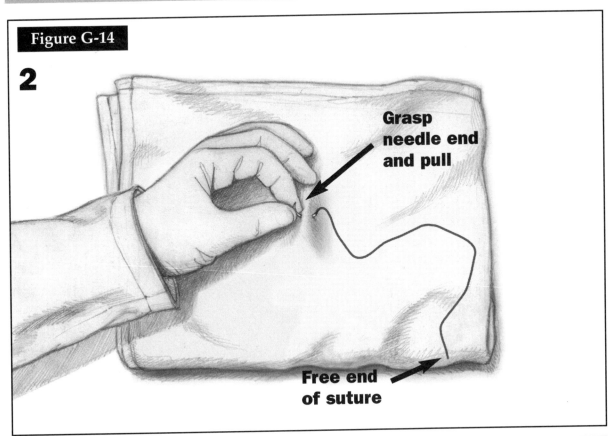

Grasp
needle end
and pull

Free end
of suture

**Figure G-14**

**3**

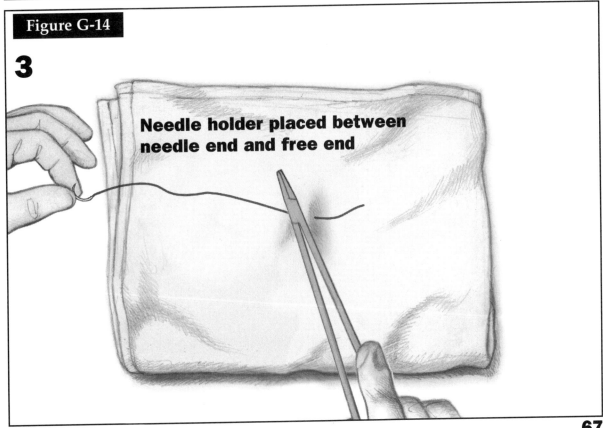

Needle holder placed between
needle end and free end

# G. Sutures and Knots

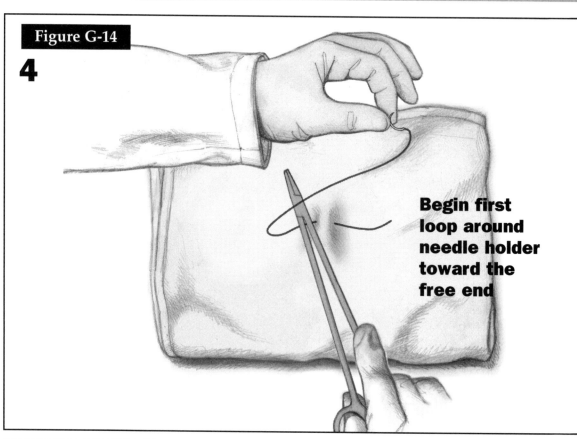

**Figure G-14**

**4**

Begin first loop around needle holder toward the free end

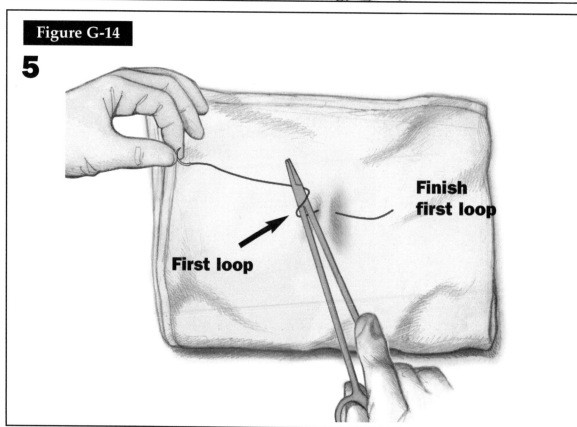

**Figure G-14**

**5**

First loop

Finish first loop

# G. Sutures and Knots

Figure G-14

**6**

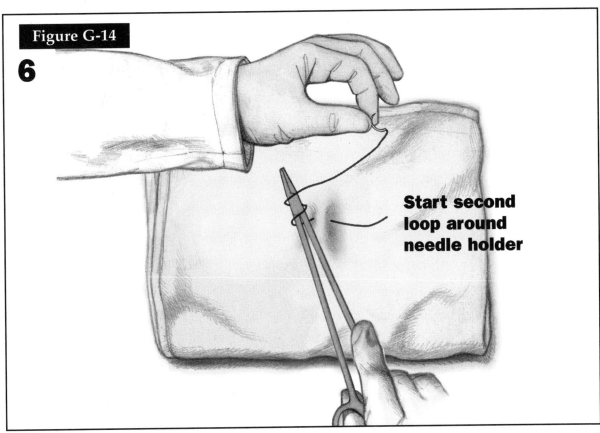

Start second loop around needle holder

Figure G-14

**7**

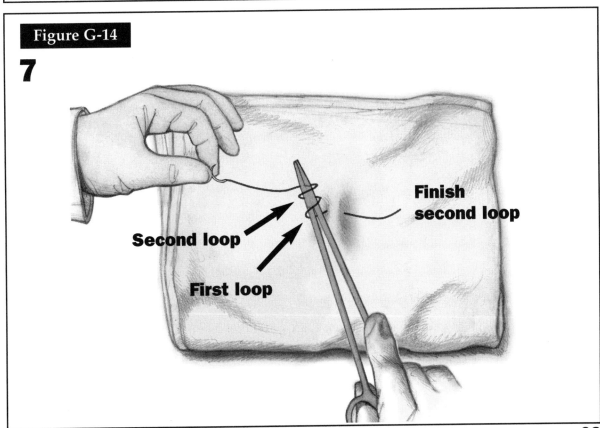

Second loop

First loop

Finish second loop

# G. Sutures and Knots

Figure G-14

**8**

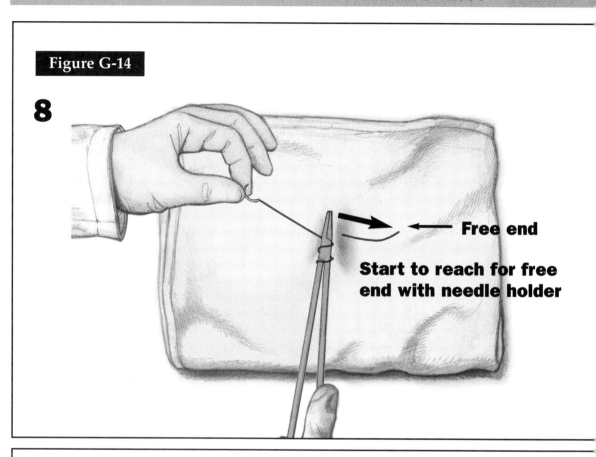

Free end

**Start to reach for free end with needle holder**

Figure G-14

**9**

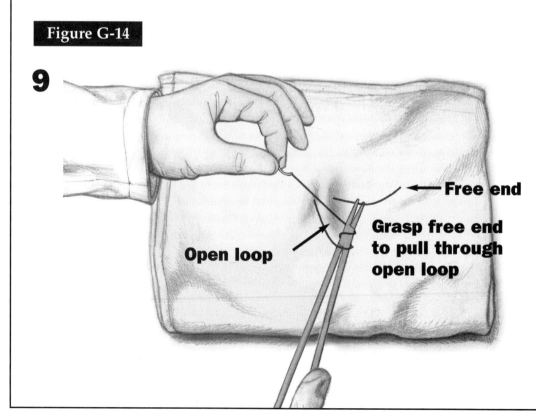

Free end

**Grasp free end to pull through open loop**

**Open loop**

# G. Sutures and Knots

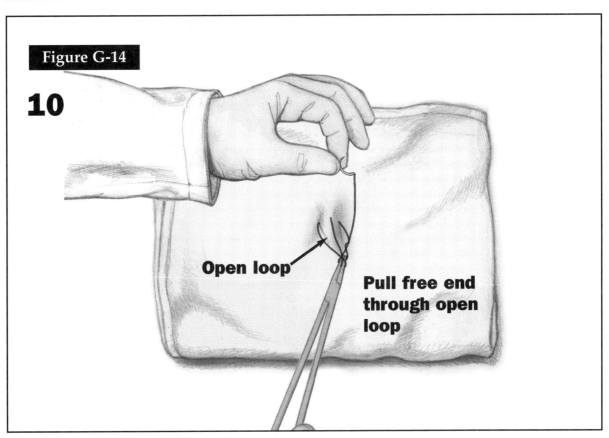

**Figure G-14**

**10**

Open loop

Pull free end through open loop

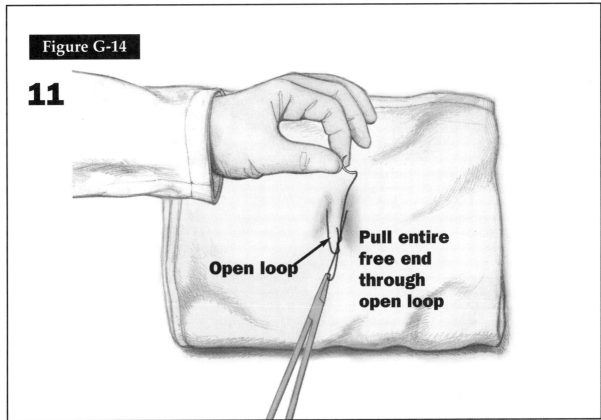

**Figure G-14**

**11**

Open loop

Pull entire free end through open loop

# G. Sutures and Knots

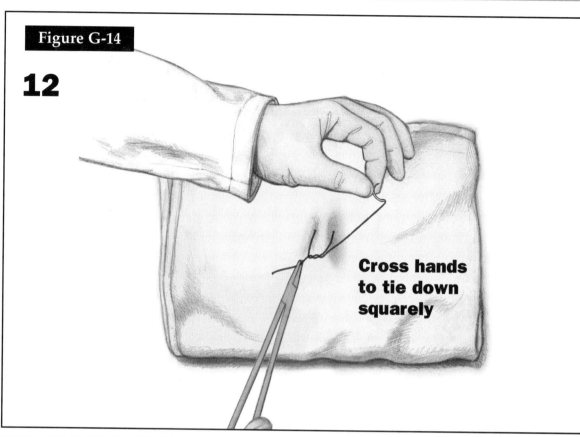

Figure G-14

**12**

Cross hands to tie down squarely

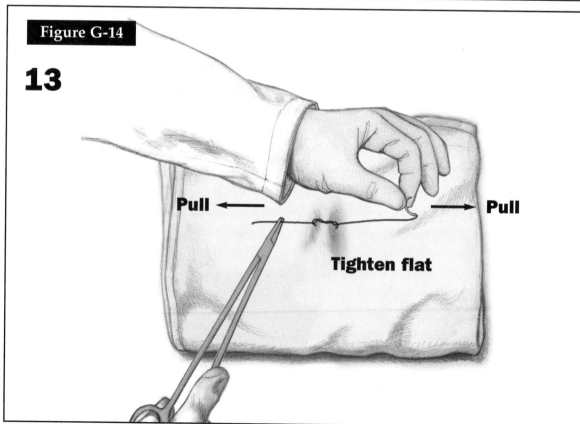

Figure G-14

**13**

Pull ← → Pull

Tighten flat

# G. Sutures and Knots

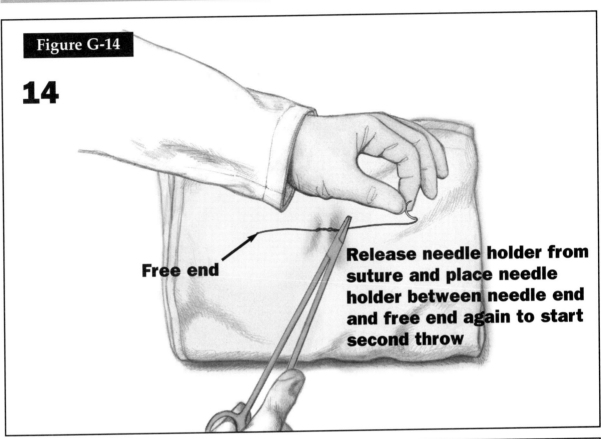

**Figure G-14**

**14**

Free end

**Release needle holder from suture and place needle holder between needle end and free end again to start second throw**

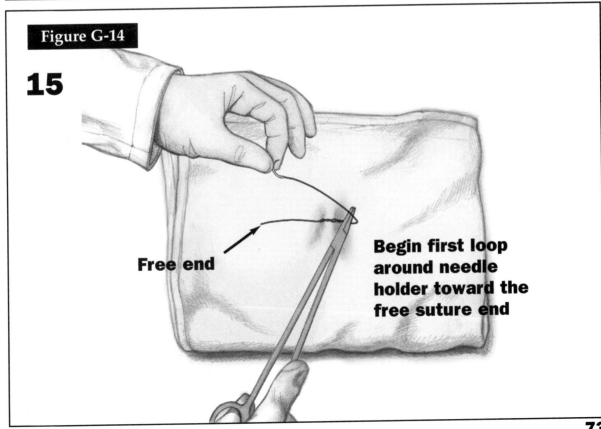

**Figure G-14**

**15**

Free end

**Begin first loop around needle holder toward the free suture end**

# G. Sutures and Knots

**Figure G-14**

**16**

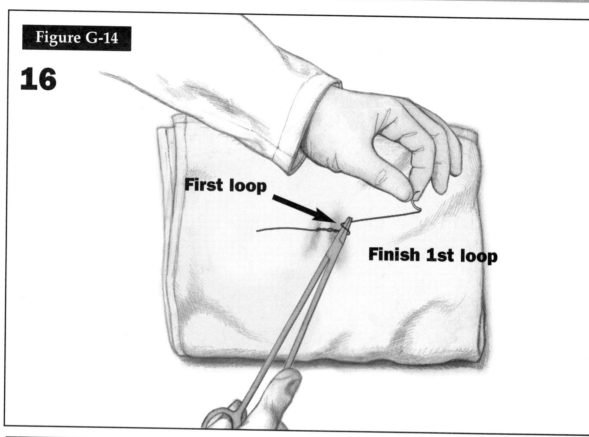

First loop

Finish 1st loop

**Figure G-14**

**17**

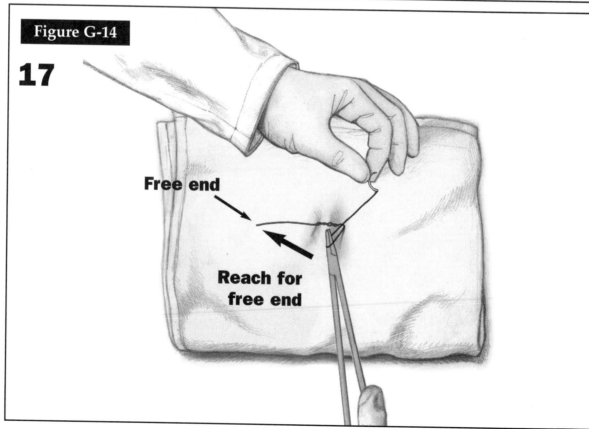

Free end

Reach for free end

# G. Sutures and Knots

**Figure G-14**

**18**

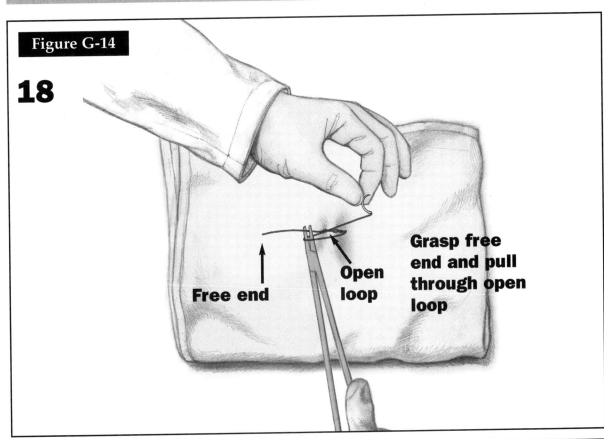

Free end

Open loop

**Grasp free end and pull through open loop**

**Figure G-14**

**19**

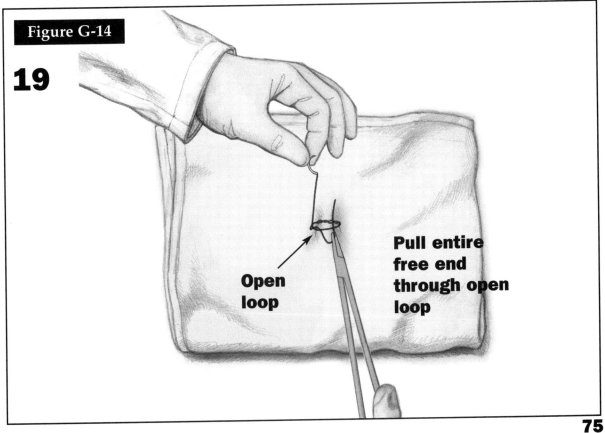

Open loop

**Pull entire free end through open loop**

# G. Sutures and Knots

**Figure G-14**

**20**

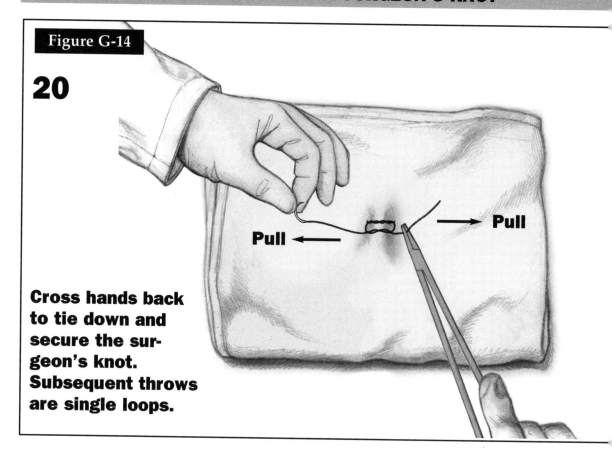

Cross hands back to tie down and secure the surgeon's knot. Subsequent throws are single loops.

# Quiz Questions

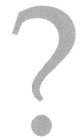

**Fill in the shaded blanks! See page 43, Table G-1 for the correct answers.**

Table G-1.
## ABSORBABLE Suture Materials

| NAME | MATERIAL | TENSILE STRENGTH | TISSUE° REACTIVITY | HANDLING† | KNOT∞ SECURITY | ABSORPTION |
|------|----------|------------------|--------------------|-----------|-----------------|------------|
| 1. COLLAGEN (plain/chromic) | Beef tendon | | | | | 1 to 2 weeks |
| 2. SURGICAL GUT (plain) | Animal collagen | | | | | 1 to 2 weeks |
| 3. SURGICAL GUT (chromic) | Animal collagen | | | | | 1 to 2 weeks |
| 4. COATED VICRYL ® | Polyglactin 910 Coated polyglactin 370 and calcium sterate | | +1 | | | 3 months |
| 5. DEXON "S" ® | Polyglycolic | | +1 | | | 3 months |
| 6. PDS ® | Polydioxanone | | +1 | | | 6 months |
| 7. MONOCRYL ® | Polyglicaprone 25 | | +1 | | | 3 months |

✷ Poor = absorbed and 0% strength by 3 weeks

✚ Good = 50% strength remains by 3 weeks

• Fair = 20% strength remains by 3 weeks

o Tendency to cause inflammation, +1 low, +4 high

† Ease of using suture

∞ Tendency to stay knotted

# H. Obtaining Hemostasis

There are a number of methods used to obtain hemostasis. These are all methods to stop bleeding. The simplest and most direct method to control bleeding is by direct finger pressure on the bleeding site. The other common methods are free vessel ligature, figure-of-eight stick tie, and electrocautery.

## 1. Free Vessel Ligature

Free vessel ligature is tying off vessels that have been clamped in a hemostat. The clamp is held by the assistant, and the surgeon passes the ligature around the hemostat. The assistant then points the tip of the hemostat facing upward. The surgeon loops the suture around the end of the hemostat so that it is encircled around the vessel. A two-hand tie of either a square knot or a surgeon's knot is then performed **(Figures H-1,2)**. After pulling down and securing the first throw of the knot, the assistant, at the surgeon's direction, releases the hemostat from the vessel. The surgeon then completes the second throw and secures the knot.

At least 4 knots should be placed in a vessel ligature unless the surgeon instructs otherwise.

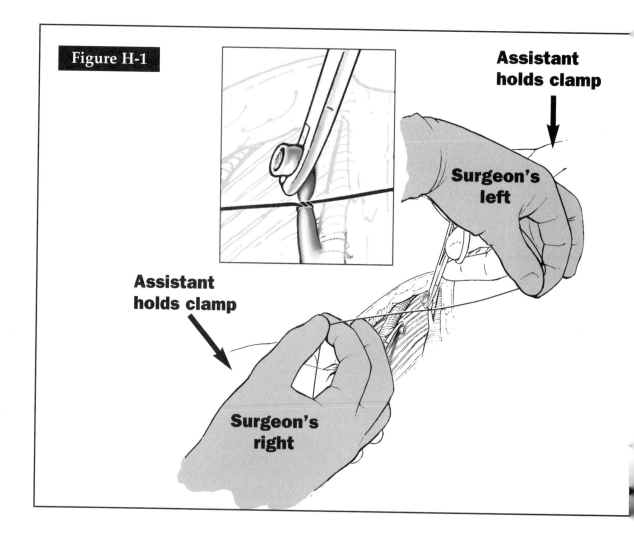

**Figure H-1**

Assistant holds clamp

Surgeon's left

Assistant holds clamp

Surgeon's right

# H. Obtaining Hemostasis

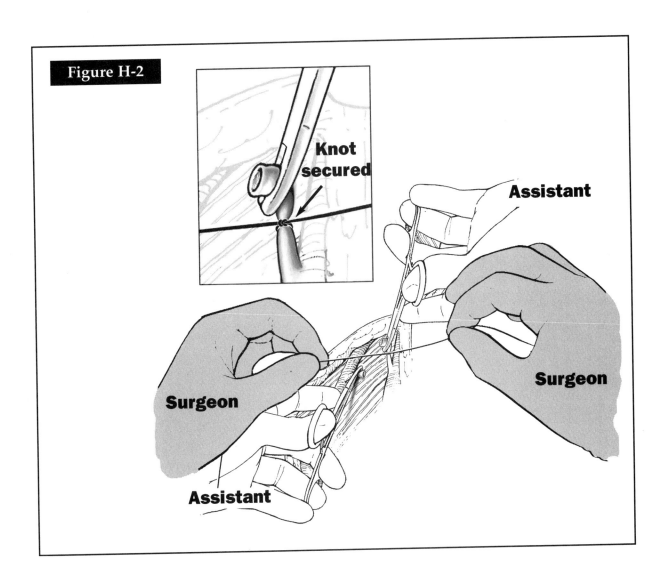

Figure H-2

Knot secured

Assistant

Surgeon

Surgeon

Assistant

# H. Obtaining Hemostasis

## 2. Figure-of-8 Stick Tie

The stick tie is a variation of the free vessel ligature and is useful for larger vessels or tissue pedicles. The stick tie is more secure and less likely to loosen and fall off during the postoperative period. The tissue to be tied is usually held in a hemostat or larger clamp. The needle is passed back and forth through the tissue under the clamp in a figure-of-8 fashion **(Figure H-3, 1-5)**

The first throw is a surgeon's knot **(Figure H-3, 6)**. The free ends of the suture are then passed around the two sides of the clamp and the knot is completed with subsequent throws **(Figure H-3, 7-12)**.

## FIGURE-OF-8 STICK TIE

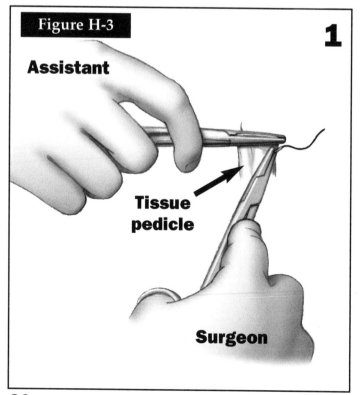

Figure H-3 **1**

Assistant

Tissue pedicle

Surgeon

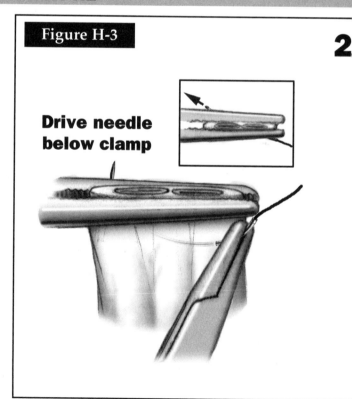

Figure H-3 **2**

Drive needle below clamp

# H. Obtaining Hemostasis

**Figure H-3** | **3**

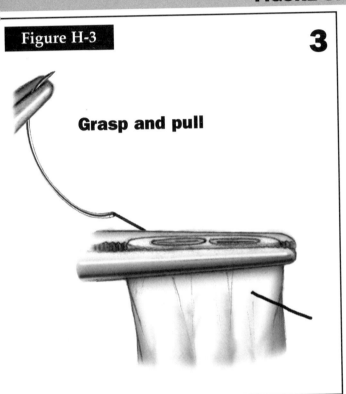

Grasp and pull

**Figure H-3** | **4**

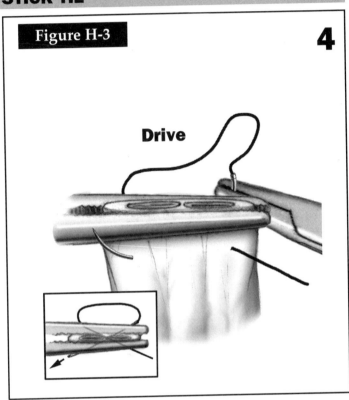

Drive

**Figure H-3** | **5**

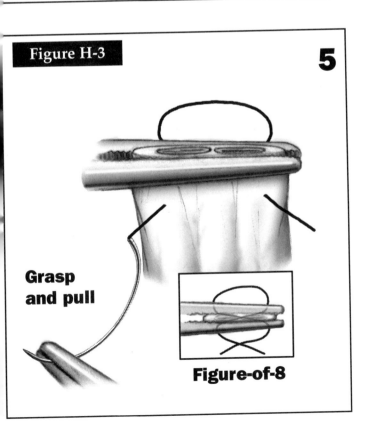

Grasp
and pull

Figure-of-8

**Figure H-3** | **6**

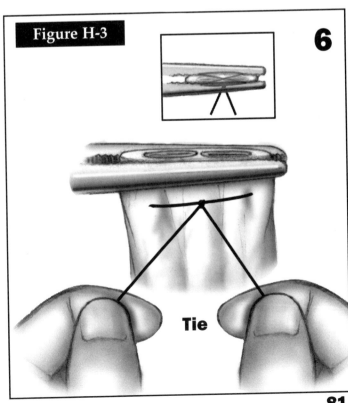

Tie

# H. Obtaining Hemostasis

**Figure H-3**    **7**

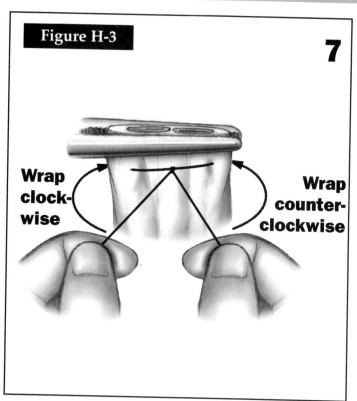

Wrap clock-wise

Wrap counter-clockwise

**Figure H-3**    **8**

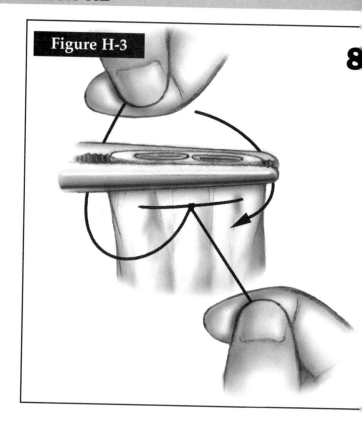

**Figure H-3**    **9**

Wrap counter-clockwise

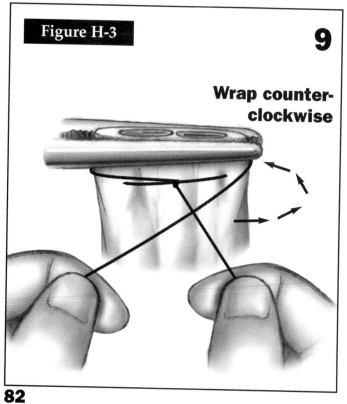

**Figure H-3**    **10**

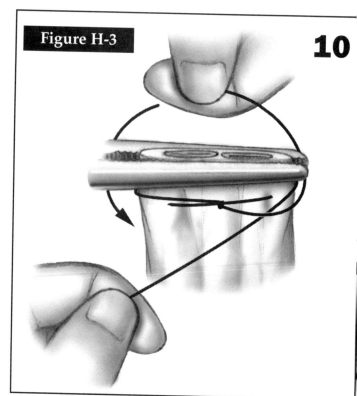

# H. Obtaining Hemostasis

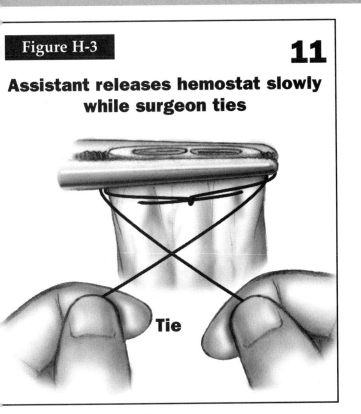

**Figure H-3** **11**

**Assistant releases hemostat slowly while surgeon ties**

Tie

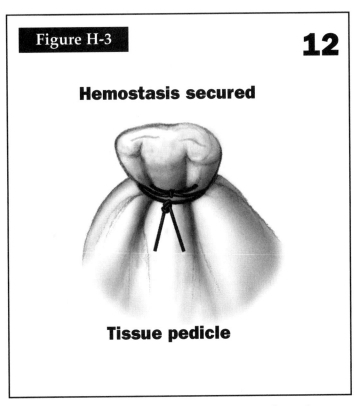

**Figure H-3** **12**

**Hemostasis secured**

**Tissue pedicle**

## 3. Electrocautery

It is faster to cauterize smaller vessels than to tie them off. The surgeon can cauterize the tiny vessels directly. Smaller vessels can also be cauterized by having the assistant hold up the clamped vessel on the hemostat. The surgeon then touches the hemostat with a monopolar cautery. This results in coagulation of the vessel. When the vessel appears adequately coagulated, the surgeon will instruct the assistant to release the hemostat from the vessel. **DO NOT RELEASE THE HEMOSTAT FROM THE VESSEL PRIOR TO DIRECTION FROM THE SURGEON**. If you do release the hemostat from the vessel prior to the coagulation, what will happen? Answer: The vessel will bleed, and the surgeon will be mighty miffed. You will learn not to do that again!

Bipolar cautery, which looks like a forceps, can be used to both grasp and cauterize bleeding vessels directly. This cautery results in burning only the tissue held between the teeth of the instrument. As previously mentioned, there is less transmission of heat and less tissue damage to the surrounding tissues with this technique. The bipolar cautery technique is excellent for stopping bleeding from smaller blood vessels.

## 4. Bone Wax

Bleeding areas of bone can usually be controlled with bone wax. This sterile material is a soft, clay-like substance that is smeared on the bleeding area to occlude the bleeding sites in bone.

# I. Wound Closure

## 1. Principles of Halving

When closing an incision, it is helpful to find the midpoint and place the first suture (central suture) at that site. The suture is placed a few millimeters back from the actual skin edge. The next sutures are then placed in halves on each side of the central suture. Thus, subsequent halving results in complete and even closure of the wound edge (**Figure I-1**). The principle of halving can be used for both deep closure and skin closure.

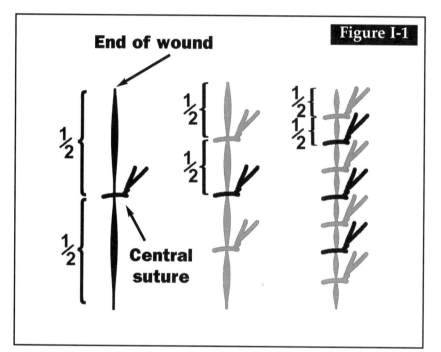

End of wound

Figure I-1

Central suture

## 2. Subcutaneous Closure

The anatomic layers of the wound are seen in **Figure I-2**. Large openings in subcutaneous tissue must be closed to prevent dead space in the wound and to take tension off the skin edge. Usually these sutures are placed so that the knots are buried. The first bite is taken away from the surface of the wound edge, deep in the wound, and the needle comes through just below the wound surface (**Figure I-3: 1-4**). The second bite goes to the opposite side at a corresponding but equal distance from the surface of the wound edge, and the needle passes deeper into the wound

(**Figure I-3: 5-8**). The knot is thus buried deep in the wound beneath the wound edge (**Figure I-3: 9,10**). This prevents extrusion of the knot through the skin.

## 3. Subcuticular Closure

In some cases the dermal (subcuticular) layer is closed in the same fashion as the subcutaneous layer, using a buried suture technique. The first bite comes away from the wound edge up into the dermis and exits the dermis just below the wound edge (**Figure I-3: 1-4**). The second bite goes in just below the wound edge on the opposite side and exits at the same distance as in the first bite (**Figure I-3: 5-8**). The knot is then tied in a buried fashion. This is similar to the subcutaneous closure, except the suture is passed through the dermal (subcuticular) layer. This takes further tension off the skin edge and assists in wound edge eversion, resulting in an improved scar in moderate to high tension wounds. Low tension wounds do not necessitate subcuticular closure in this manner.

## 4. Skin Closure

Once the appropriate subcutaneous and dermal (subcuticular) closures have been done, it is time to close the cut epidermal (skin) layer (**Figure I-3: 11,12**). A variety of techniques are available to close the incised skin edges. Each technique is designed to accomplish the same things: to decrease tension at the epidermal edge during healing, to precisely oppose the skin edges so as to produce the least amount of trauma to the surrounding soft tissues, and to prevent wound infection by direct contamination. All of this promotes healing and will result in a less conspicuous scar.

# I. Wound Closure

Figure I-2

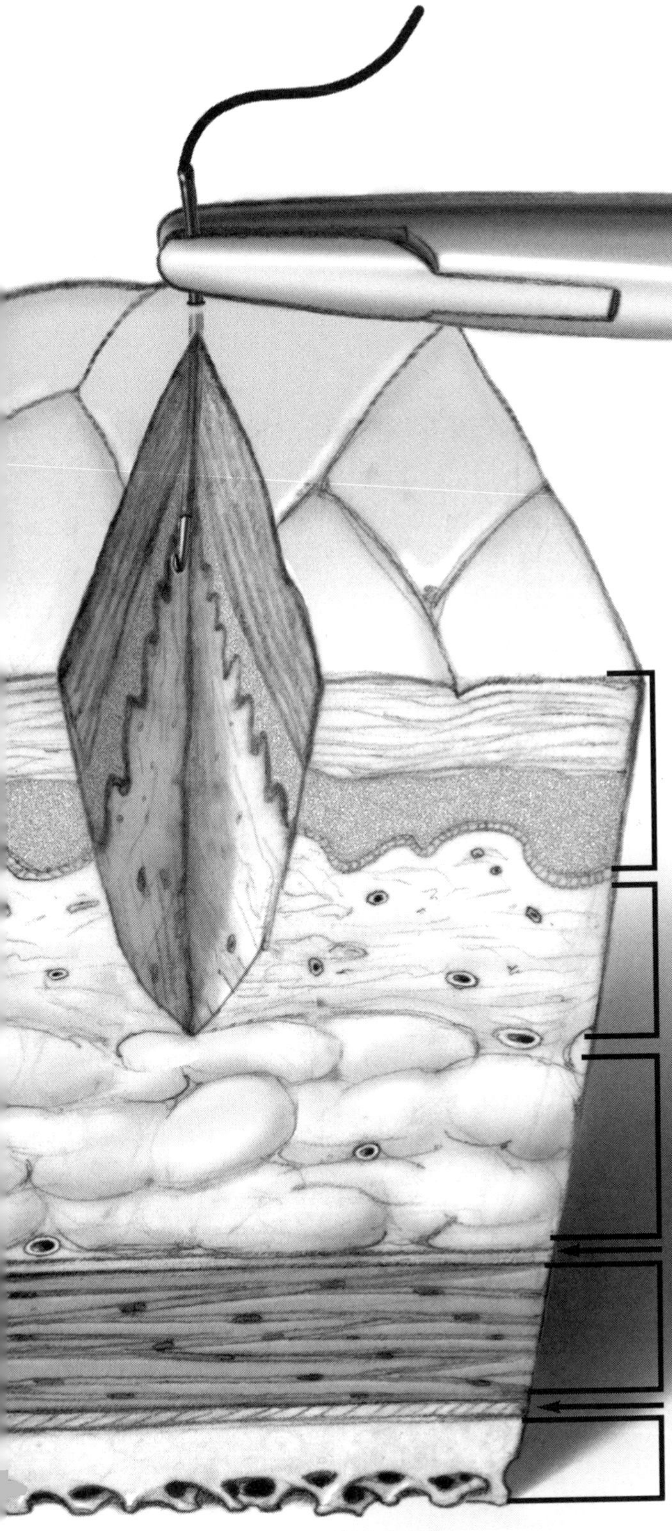

**ANATOMICAL STRUCTURE**

**SUTURE LOCATION AND TERMS**

A. **SKIN**
  1. **Epidermis**

1. **SKIN SUTURE**
   a. Epidermis alone or
   b. Epidermis and dermis

  2. **Dermis**

2. **INTRADERMAL SUTURE**
   (also called subcuticular or intracuticular suture)
   1. Dermis only

B. **SUBCUTANEOUS TISSUE** (fat and connective tissue)

3. **SUBCUTANEOUS SUTURE**
   1. Subcutaneous tissue

C. **FASCIA**

4. **FASCIAL SUTURE**
   1. Fascia only

D. **MUSCLE**

5. **MUSCLE SUTURE**
   1. Muscle only

E. **PERIOSTEUM**

6. **PERIOSTEUM**
   1. Periosteum only

F. **BONE**

# I. Wound Closure

### Figure I-3

**1**

## INCORRECT
## wound closure

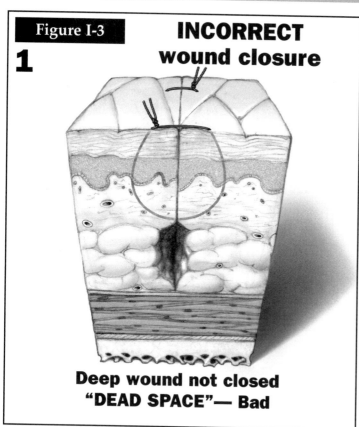

**Deep wound not closed
"DEAD SPACE"— Bad**

### Figure I-3

**2**

## CORRECT
## deep wound closure

**Start first
bite "low"**

**Enter
wound
"low"**

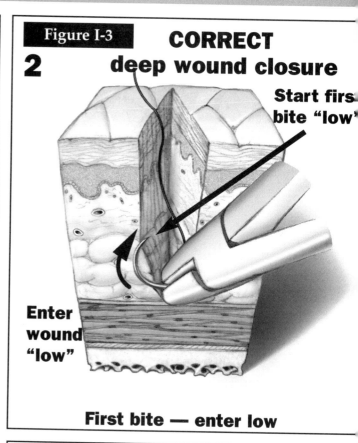

**First bite — enter low**

### Figure I-3

**3**

**Grasp
and pull**

**Exit
"high"**

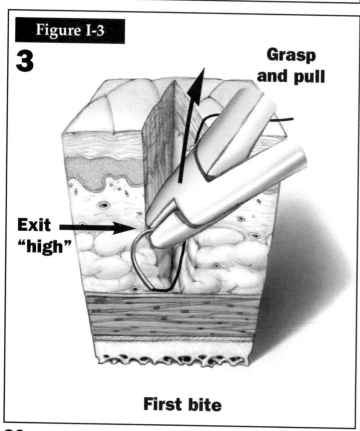

**First bite**

### Figure I-3

**4**

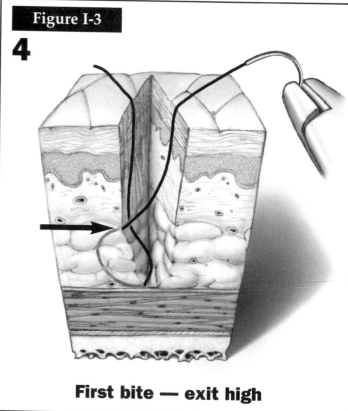

**First bite — exit high**

# I. Wound Closure

**Figure I-3**

**5** **Drive**

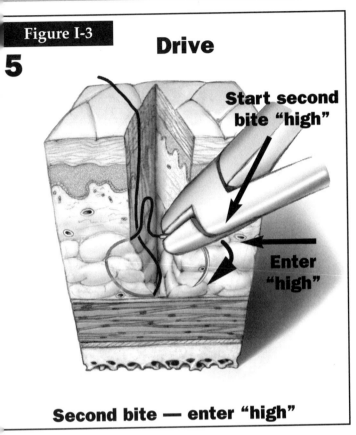

Start second bite "high"

Enter "high"

**Second bite — enter "high"**

**Figure I-3**

**6** **Grasp and pull**

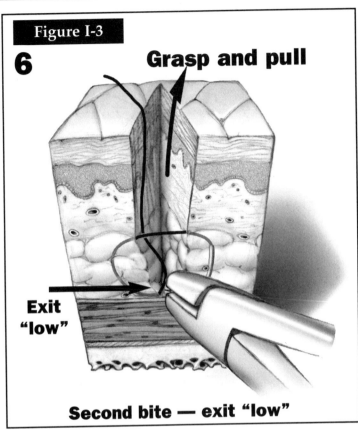

Exit "low"

**Second bite — exit "low"**

**Figure I-3**

**7** **Tie**

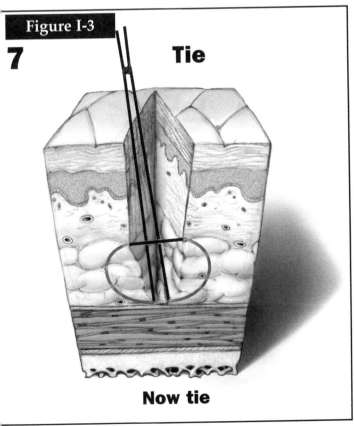

**Now tie**

**Figure I-3**

**8**

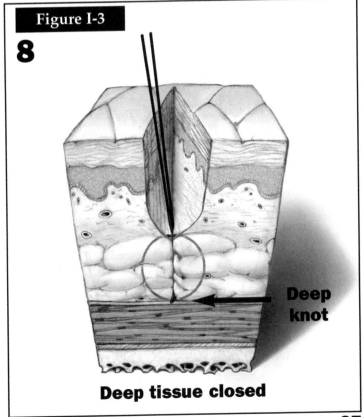

Deep knot

**Deep tissue closed**

# I. Wound Closure

## DEEP WOUND CLOSURE

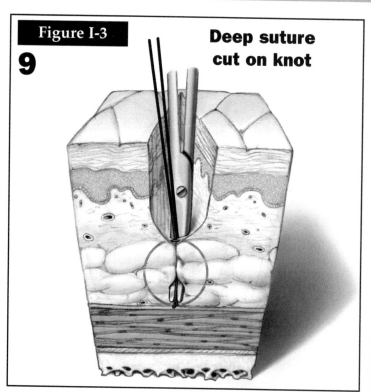

**Figure I-3**

**9**

Deep suture
cut on knot

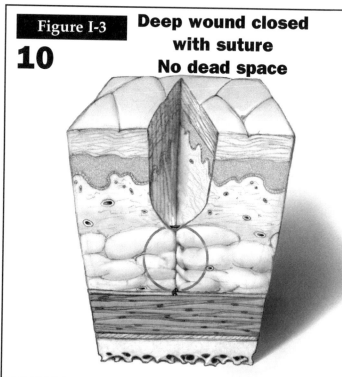

**Figure I-3**

**10**

Deep wound closed
with suture
No dead space

## SKIN CLOSURE

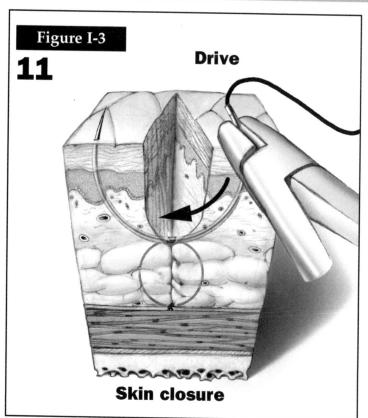

**Figure I-3**

**11**

Drive

Skin closure

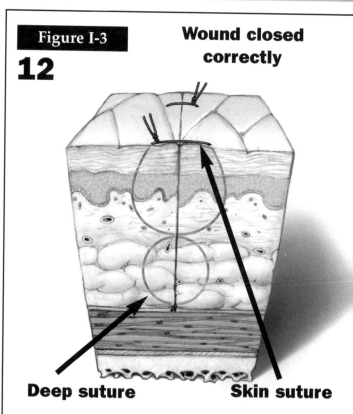

**Figure I-3**

**12**

Wound closed
correctly

Deep suture     Skin suture

# Quiz Questions

Fill in the shaded blanks! See page 85, Figure I-2 for the correct answers.

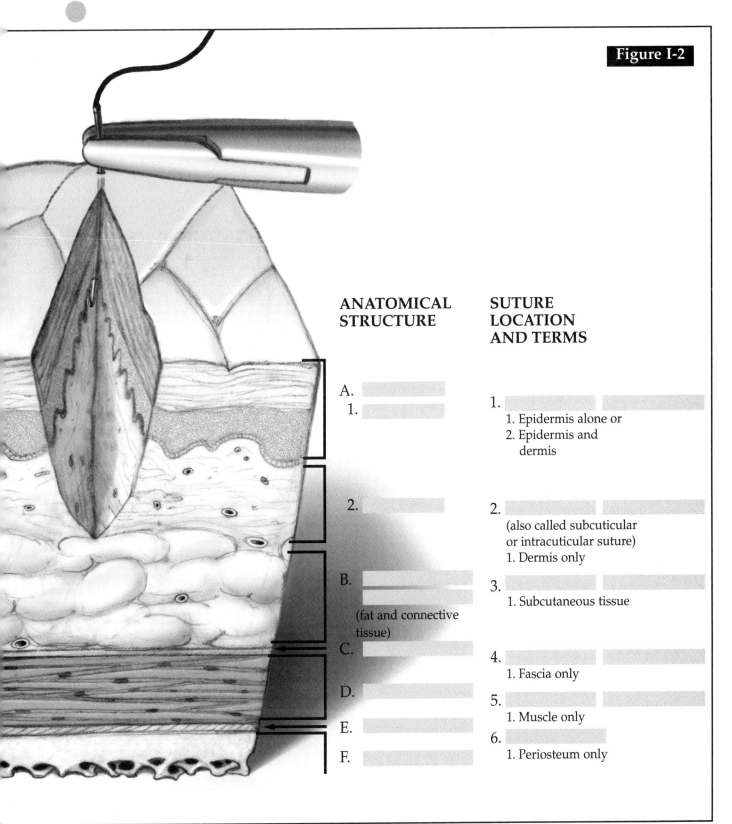

Figure I-2

**ANATOMICAL STRUCTURE**

A. ▢
  1. ▢

2. ▢

B. ▢

(fat and connective tissue)

C. ▢

D. ▢

E. ▢

F. ▢

**SUTURE LOCATION AND TERMS**

1. ▢ ▢
   1. Epidermis alone or
   2. Epidermis and dermis

2. ▢ ▢
   (also called subcuticular or intracuticular suture)
   1. Dermis only

3. ▢ ▢
   1. Subcutaneous tissue

4. ▢ ▢
   1. Fascia only

5. ▢ ▢
   1. Muscle only

6. ▢
   1. Periosteum only

# I. Wound Closure

### a. Simple Interrupted Suture

The simple interrupted suture is one of the most commonly used suture techniques. These sutures are useful in essentially any situation. It is a one-bite suture technique. The needle is passed through the skin **PERPENDICULAR** to the skin edge (**Figure I-4**). The needle passes through the entire epidermis and dermis. The second portion of the bite comes out through the opposite side at the same distance from the wound edge and tied (**Figure I-5,6**). The goal is to approximate and evert the wound edge. The drawings show the technique of the simple interrupted suture (**Figure I-7**). Note the incorrect and correct (**PERPENDICULAR**) angle of approach to the skin surface. The **PERPENDICULAR** angle of approach helps to evert the wound edges.

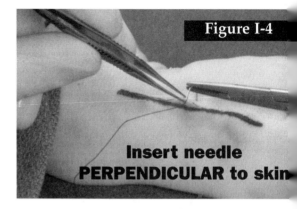

Figure I-4

**Insert needle
PERPENDICULAR to skin**

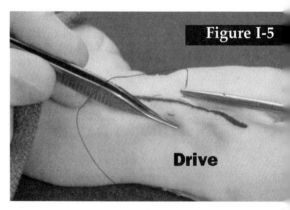

Figure I-5

**Drive**

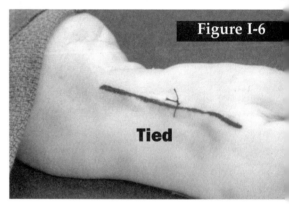

Figure I-6

**Tied**

# I. Wound Closure

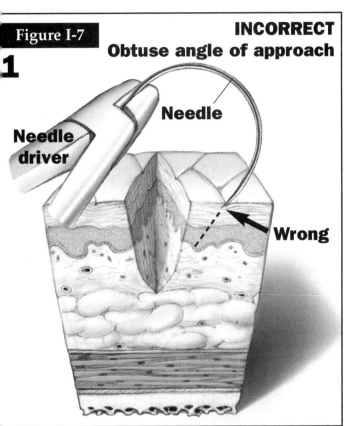

**Figure I-7**

**1**

**INCORRECT**
**Obtuse angle of approach**

Needle

Needle driver

Wrong

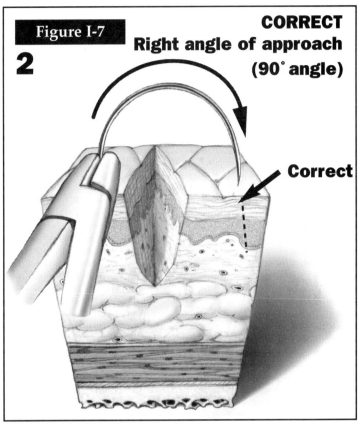

**Figure I-7**

**2**

**CORRECT**
**Right angle of approach**
**(90° angle)**

Correct

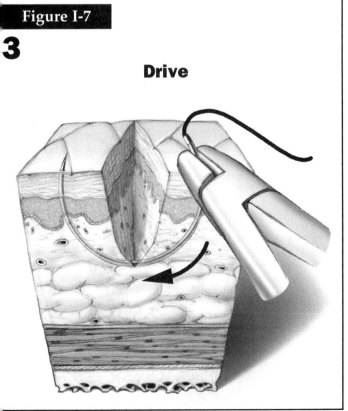

**Figure I-7**

**3**

Drive

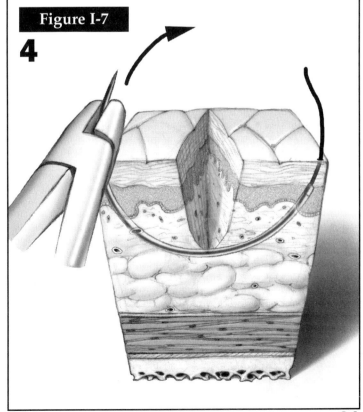

**Figure I-7**

**4**

# I. Wound Closure

### Figure I-7

**5**

Tie

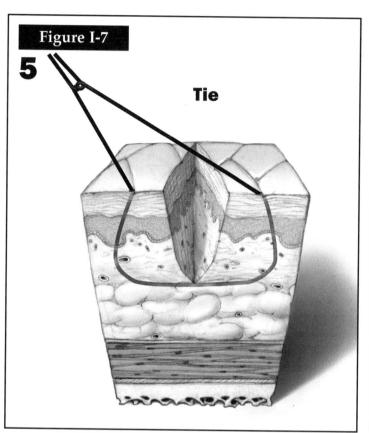

### Figure I-7

**6**

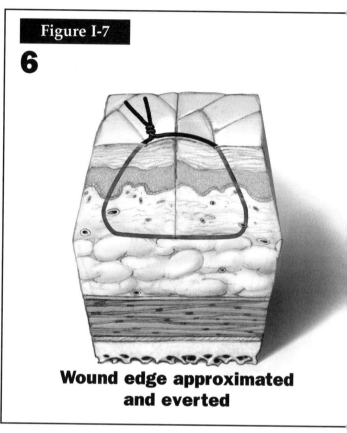

**Wound edge approximated
and everted**

### Figure I-7

**7**

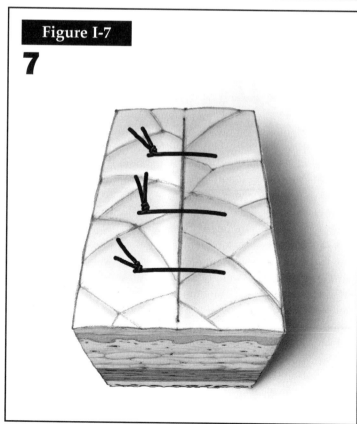

# Quiz Questions

Fill in the shaded blanks! See page 91, Figure I-7 for the correct answers.

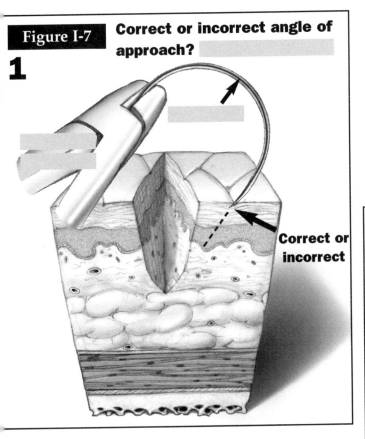

**Figure I-7**

**1**

Correct or incorrect angle of approach?

Correct or incorrect

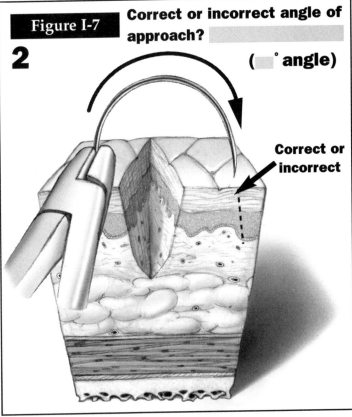

**Figure I-7**

**2**

Correct or incorrect angle of approach?

(       ° angle)

Correct or incorrect

# I. Wound Closure

### b. Vertical Mattress Suture

The vertical mattress is a two-bite suture technique. The bites closer to the cut edge of the wound are utilized to precisely oppose and evert the skin edges. The vertical mattress suture is useful when the tissues tend to invert with placement of simple sutures. The vertical mattress gives both excellent eversion and precise skin edge apposition.

The first small bites are placed 1 to 2 mm from the cut edge of wound at the intradermal level **(Figure I-8)**. After the first small bite is precisely placed, the two portions of the suture on each side of the incision are grasped and pulled up **(Figure I-9)**. This provides automatic eversion of the tissue before the next deeper bite. The deeper (second) bite is then placed away from the skin edge starting on the same side of the needle and coming back to the starting side where the free end of the suture is located **(Figure I-10)**.

The suture is then tied on the side of the wound where the wound closure first started **(Figure I-11)**. The deeper second bite helps reduce tension from the wound edge while the shorter first bite precisely matches the skin edges. The resultant eversion with this suturing technique is excellent and provides less risk of hypertrophic scarring. The drawings show the technical details of the vertical mattress suture **(Figure I-12, 1-6)**.

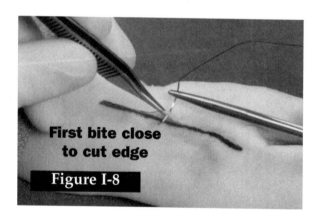

First bite close to cut edge

**Figure I-8**

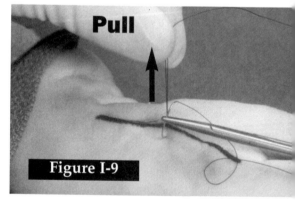

Pull

**Figure I-9**

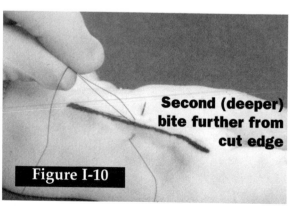

Second (deeper) bite further from cut edge

**Figure I-10**

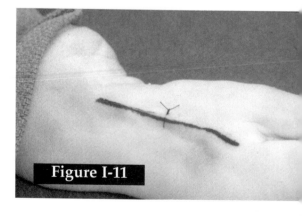

**Figure I-11**

# I. Wound Closure

Figure I-12 **1**

**First bite close to cut edge**

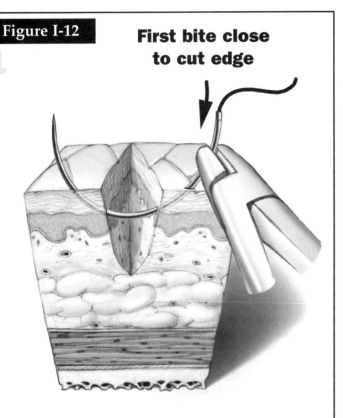

Figure I-12 **2**

**Grasp and pull**

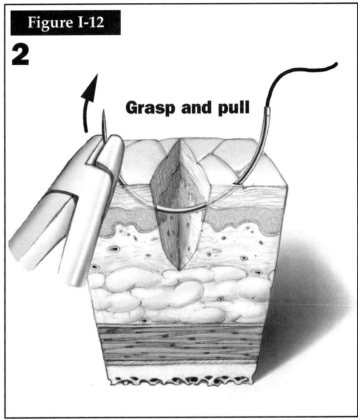

Figure I-12 **3**

**Pull**

**Free end**

**Second bite further from cut edge**

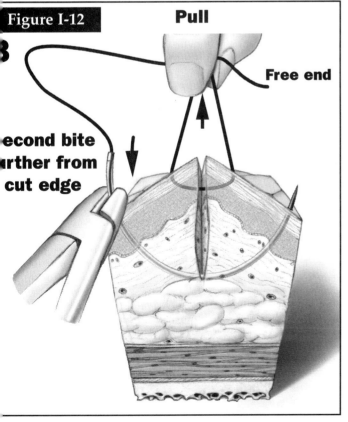

Figure I-12 **4**

**Grasp and pull**

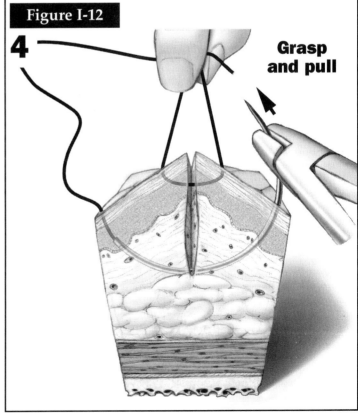

# I. Wound Closure

**Figure I-12**

## 5

**Tie**

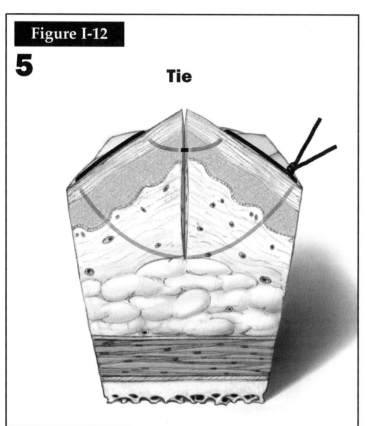

**Figure I-12**

## 6

# Vertical mattress

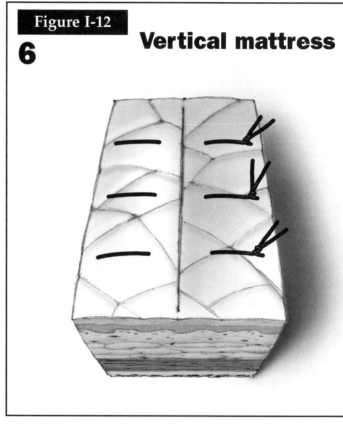

# *Quiz Questions*

Fill in the shaded blanks!
See page 29, Figure F-6 for the correct answers.

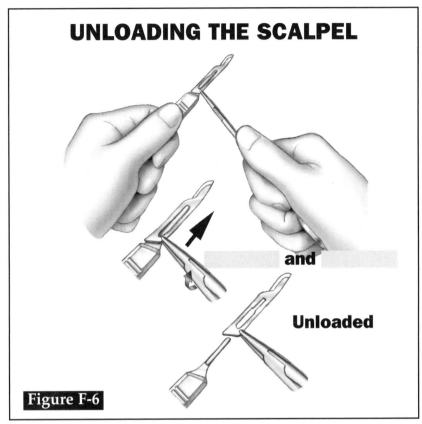

**UNLOADING THE SCALPEL**

and

**Unloaded**

Figure F-6

See page 38, Figure F-28 for the correct answers.

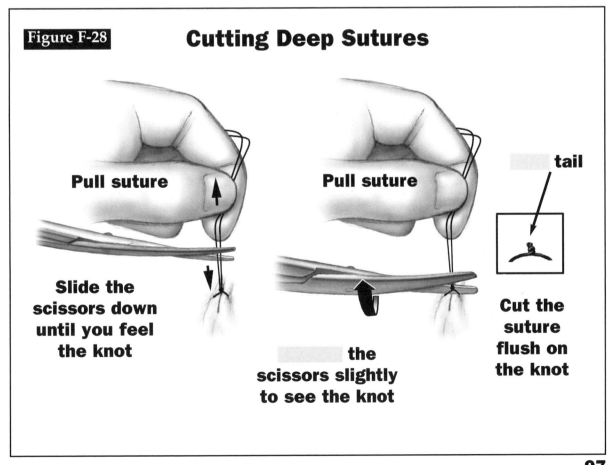

Figure F-28

**Cutting Deep Sutures**

Pull suture

Slide the scissors down until you feel the knot

Pull suture

the scissors slightly to see the knot

tail

Cut the suture flush on the knot

# I. Wound Closure

### c. Horizontal Mattress Suture

The horizontal mattress suture is also a two-bite suture technique. These two bites are parallel to each other on each side of the wound. The horizontal mattress everts tissue well but does not bring the skin edges precisely together in all cases. Sometimes wide horizontal mattress sutures are placed to evert the epidermis and take tension off the wound edge. Then a few small simple interrupted sutures or steri-strips are placed at the skin edge to precisely close and approximate the cut wound edges. The horizontal mattress everts as well as the vertical mattress, but is faster to place. The first bite is done exactly as the simple suture **(Figure I-13)**. The second bite is done parallel to the first bite and goes back across the wound edge to end on the same side as the first bite **(Figure I-14)**. The suture is tied on the side of the first bite **(Figure I-15)**. The drawings show the technical details of the horizontal mattress **(Figure I-16, 1-6)**. In both the vertical mattress suture technique and the horizontal mattress suture technique, no suture externally crosses the cut edge of the wound.

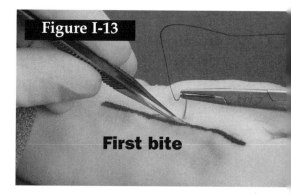

**Figure I-13**

**First bite**

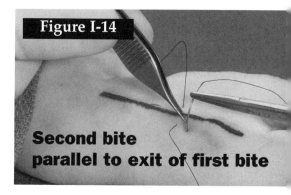

**Figure I-14**

**Second bite parallel to exit of first bite**

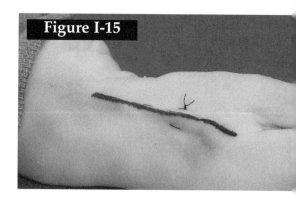

**Figure I-15**

# I. Wound Closure

## HORIZONTAL MATTRESS SUTURE

**Figure I-16**

**1** Drive

Free end ↓

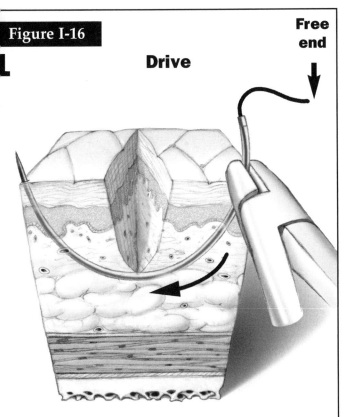

**Figure I-16**

**2** Grasp and pull

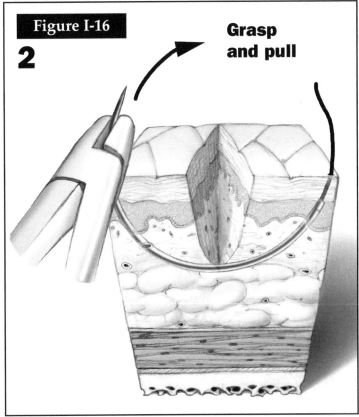

**Figure I-16**

**3** Drive

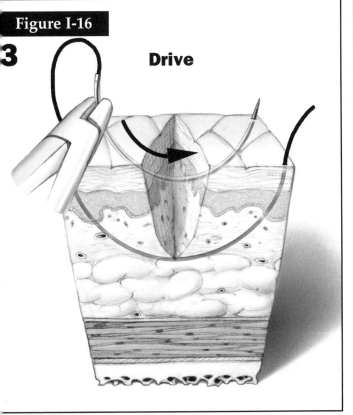

**Figure I-16**

**4** Grasp and pull

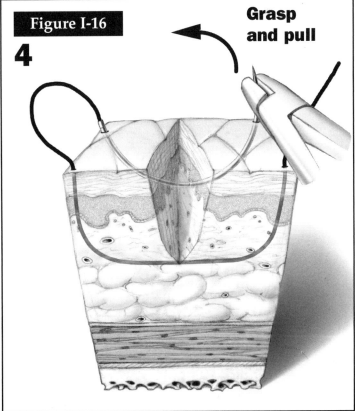

## HORIZONTAL MATTRESS SUTURE

**Figure I-16**

**5**    Tie

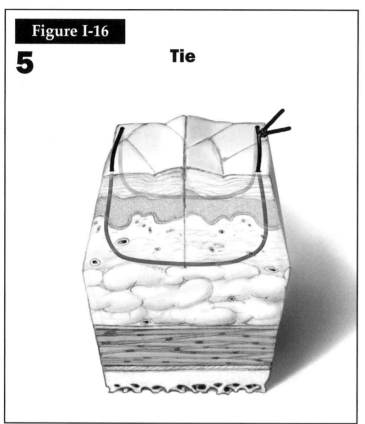

**Figure I-16**

**6**    Horizontal mattress

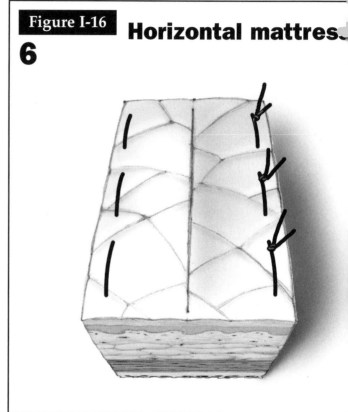

# Quiz Questions

Fill in the shaded blanks! See page 99, Figure I-16 for the correct answers.
This is a Horizontal Mattress Suture.

**Figure I-16**

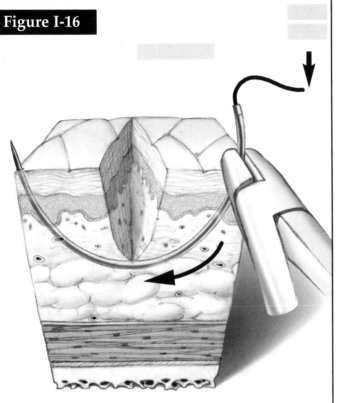

**Figure I-16**

**2**

&

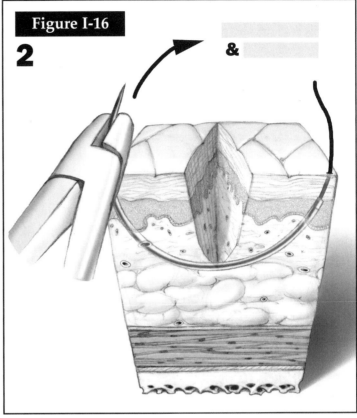

**Figure I-16**

**3**

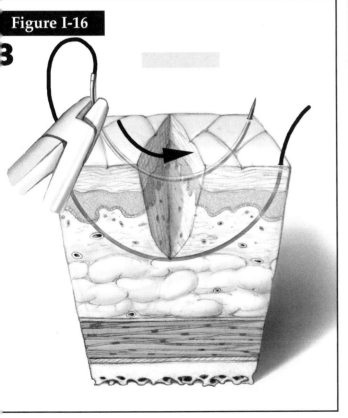

**Figure I-16**

**4**

&

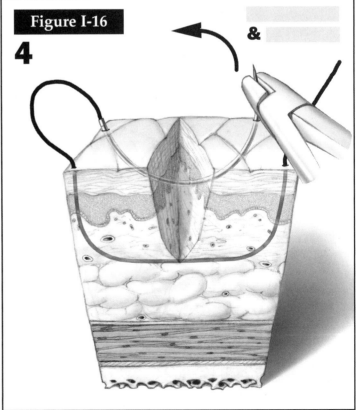

### d. Running Closure ("Baseball Stitch")

The running closure is often used when the wound's edges easily evert and a long straight incision needs closing. If there is a significant risk of hematoma, the running closure should not be used for the entire length of the incision, as all of the sutures would have to be removed to drain the hematoma.

If simple interrupted sutures are placed n[ear] the ends of the wound, then only these int[er]rupted sutures need be removed for the drainage of a hematoma. The simple running closure or "baseball stitch" is started with a simple suture which is tied off **(Figure I-17)**. The free end is trimmed 3 t[o] mm to leave a tail. The end of the suture attached to the needle is not cut. The sutu[r]ing is now advanced in an equal distance along the cut edge of the wound. The nee[dle] "bites" are still perpendicular to the skin edge but the sutures cross the wound exte[r]nally. Additional simple sutures are place[d] without tying or cutting the sutures **(Figu[re] I-18, 19)**. Constant tension is held on the suture behind the next throw to prevent loosening of the previous sutures. This results in a continuous "baseball stitch" cl[o]sure.

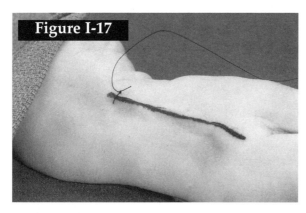

**Figure I-17**

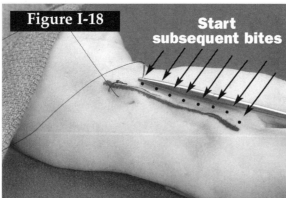

**Figure I-18**

**Start subsequent bites**

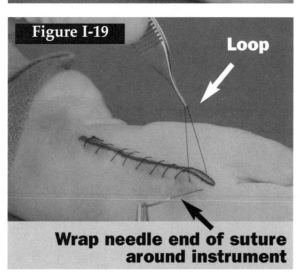

**Figure I-19**

**Loop**

**Wrap needle end of suture around instrument**

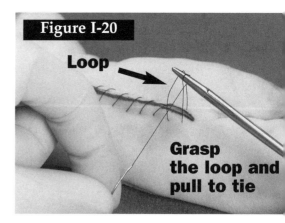

**Figure I-20**

**Loop**

**Grasp the loop and pull to tie**

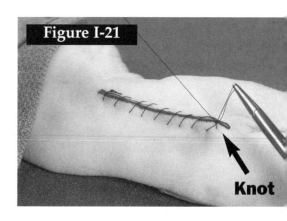

**Figure I-21**

**Knot**

# I. Wound Closure

At the end, the final throw is placed but not pulled entirely through **(Figure I-19)**. The loop on the next to last throw is utilized as a single strand and the tie done to the loop end of the suture **(Figures I-19, 20, 21)** The free strands are then cut, resulting in 3 tails. Running sutures can be removed by grasping and snipping each subsequent suture and pulling through.

The drawings show the technical details of the running closure **(Figure I-22, 1-11)**.

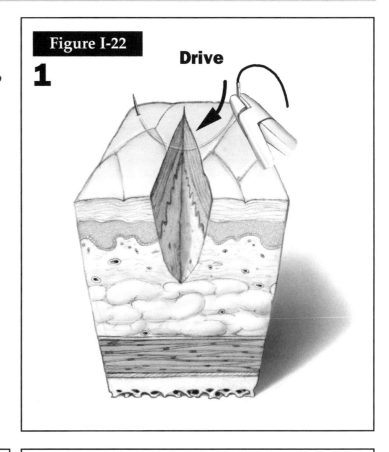

**Figure I-22**

**1**

**Drive**

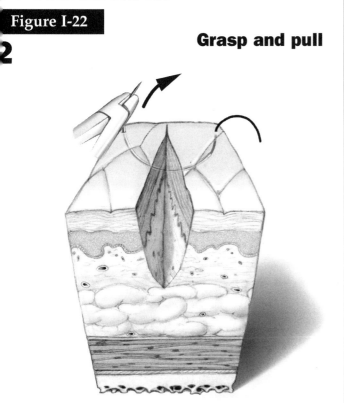

**Figure I-22**

**2**

**Grasp and pull**

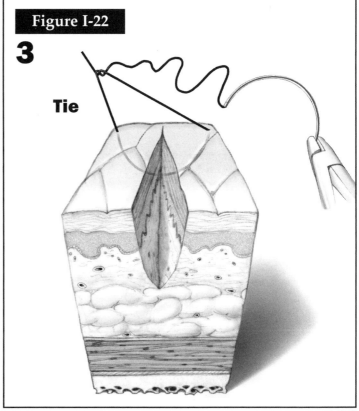

**Figure I-22**

**3**

**Tie**

# I. Wound Closure

**Figure I-22**

**4**

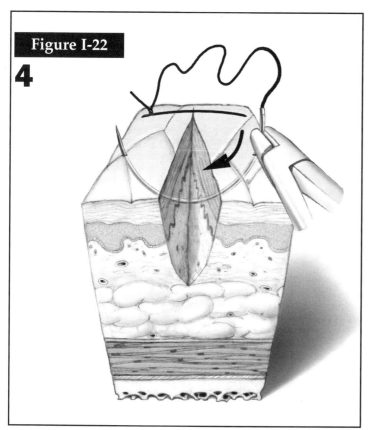

**Figure I-22**

**5**

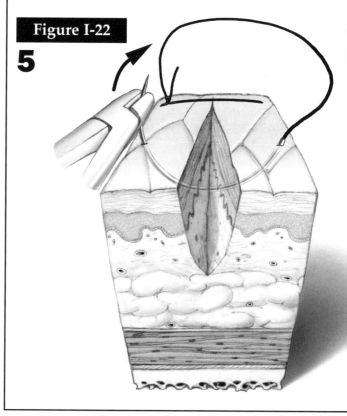

**Figure I-22**

**6**

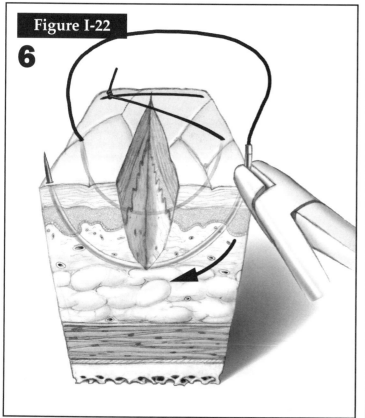

**Figure I-22**

**7**

**Grasp and pull**

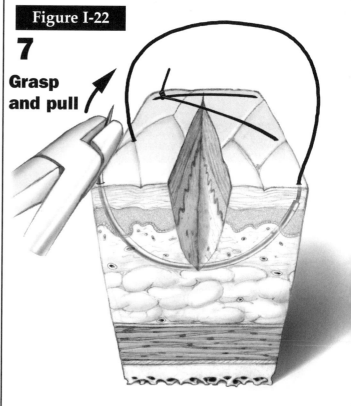

# I. Wound Closure

**Figure I-22**

**8**

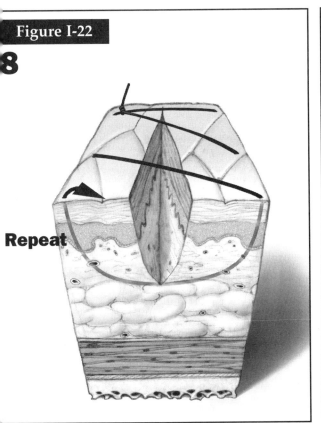

**Repeat**

**Figure I-22**

**9**

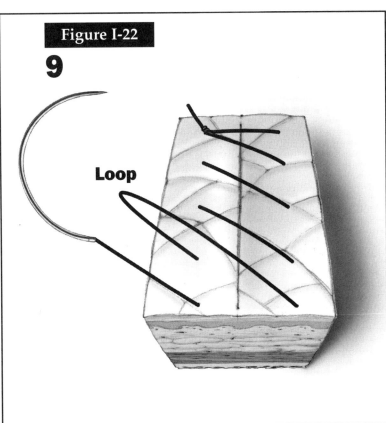

**Loop**

**Figure I-22**

**10**

**Tie the loop with the single end**

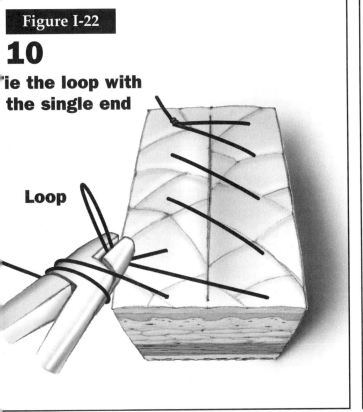

**Loop**

**Figure I-22**

**11**

**Start**

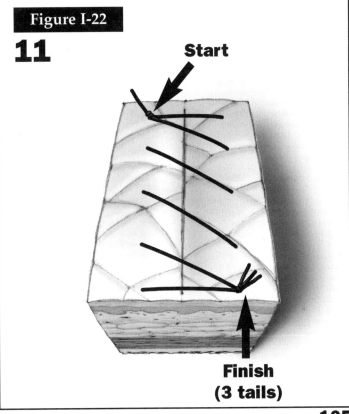

**Finish (3 tails)**

# I. Wound Closure

### e. Running-Lock Closure

The running-lock closure is a variation of the simple running closure or "baseball stitch." With this technique, the suture is LOCKED prior to placement of the next simple suture **(Figures I-24, 25)**. This results in significantly more tissue eversion. This technique also reduces the skin tension more than the running closure. Thus, in cases where the wound edges tend to invert during closure, or where there is moderate tension, a running-lock closure is a better choice than a simple running closure. In addition, it is easier to remove, as the interdigitations can each be cut away from the cut wound edge. The first and last tie are the same as in the simple running closure **(Figure I-26)**. The drawings show the technical details of the running-lock closure **(Figure I-27, 1-11 )**.

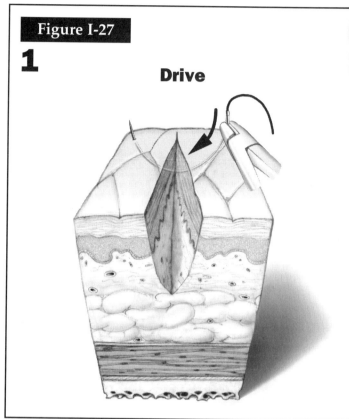

Figure I-27

**1**

**Drive**

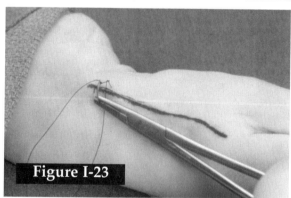

Figure I-23

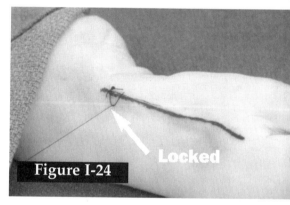

Figure I-24

**Locked**

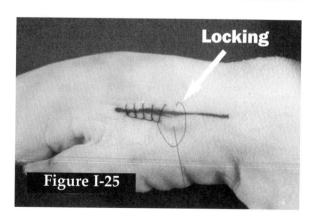

**Locking**

Figure I-25

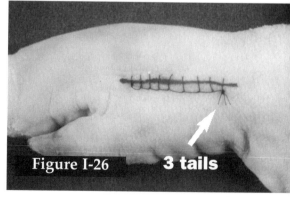

Figure I-26   **3 tails**

# I. Wound Closure

Figure I-27

**2**

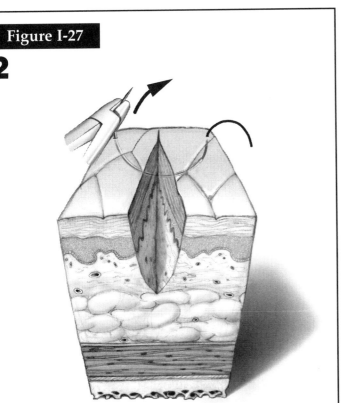

Figure I-27

**3**

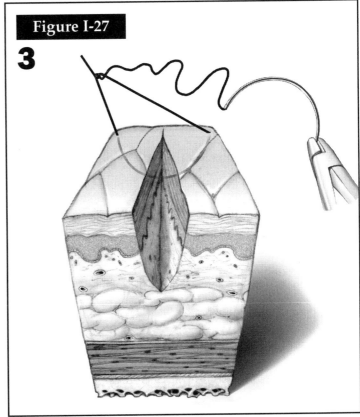

Figure I-27

**4**

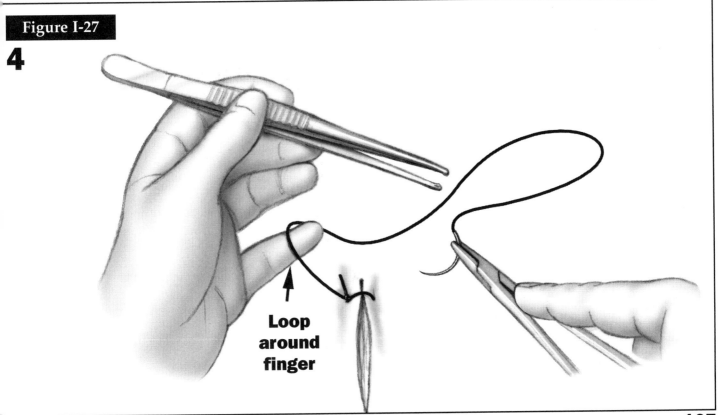

**Loop around finger**

# I. Wound Closure

**Figure I-27**

**5**

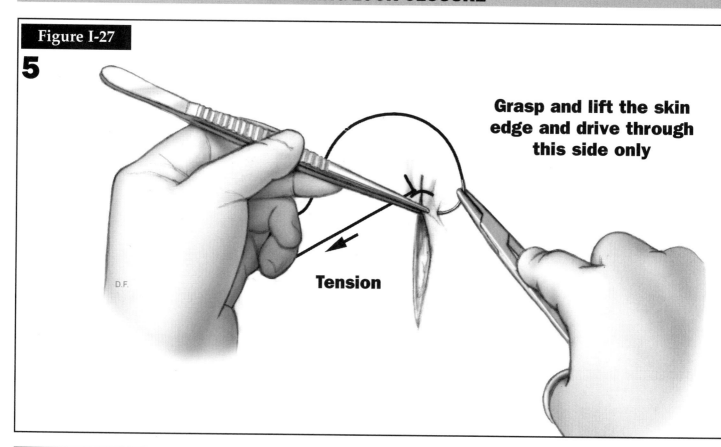

Grasp and lift the skin edge and drive through this side only

Tension

**Figure I-27**

**6**

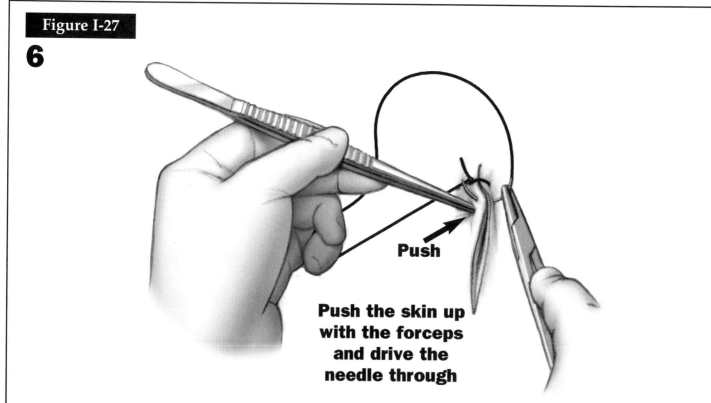

Push

Push the skin up with the forceps and drive the needle through

# I. Wound Closure

**Figure I-27**

## 7

**Bring the loop down over the needle**

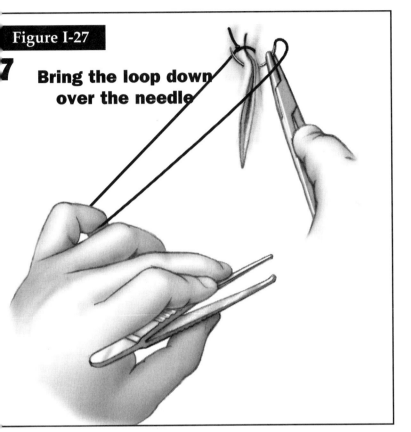

**Figure I-27**

## 8

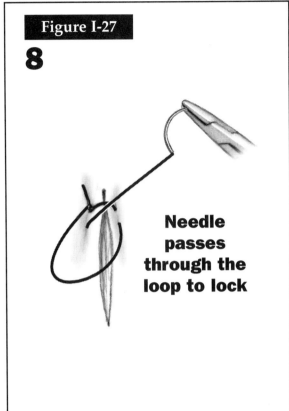

**Needle passes through the loop to lock**

**Figure I-27**

## 9

**Repeat steps 4-8**

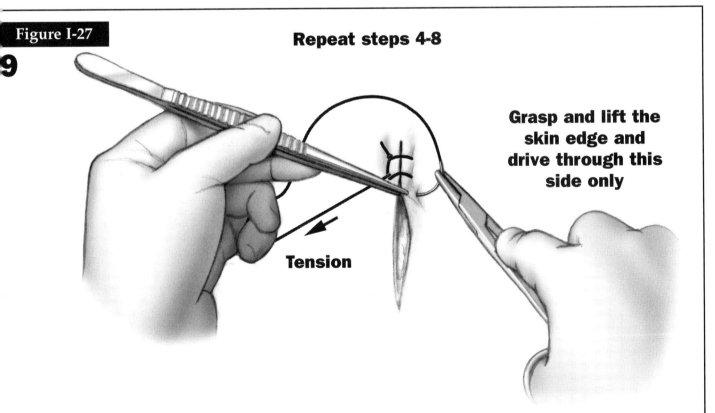

**Grasp and lift the skin edge and drive through this side only**

**Tension**

# I. Wound Closure

**Figure I-27**

## 10

Wrap needle end of suture around needle driver, grasp loop and pull to tie

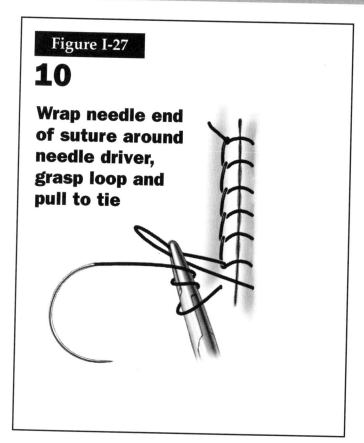

**Figure I-27**

## 11

**Running lock**

Finish (3 tails)

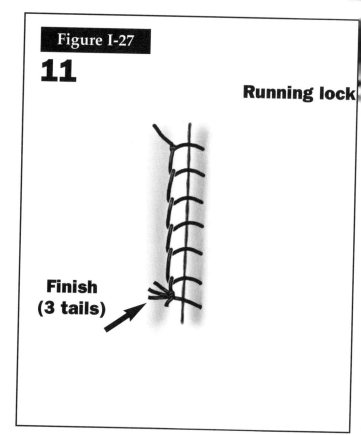

110

# Quiz

Fill in the shaded blanks! See page 105, Figure I-22 for the correct answers. This is a Running Closure.

Figure I-22

**8**

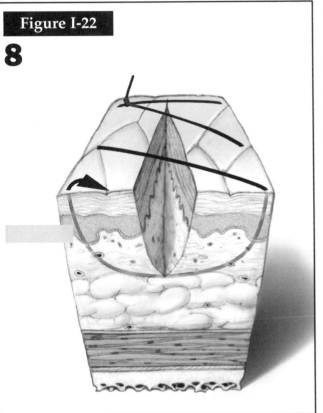

Figure I-22

**9**

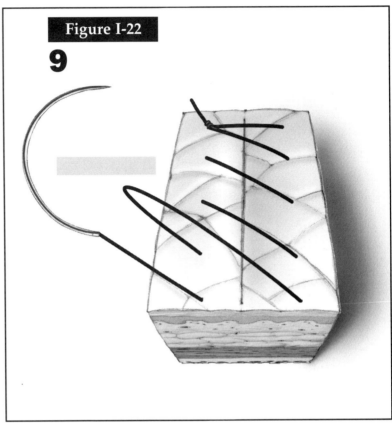

Figure I-22

**10**

the loop with
the       end

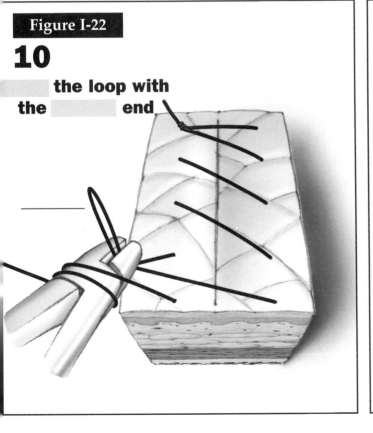

Figure I-22

**11**

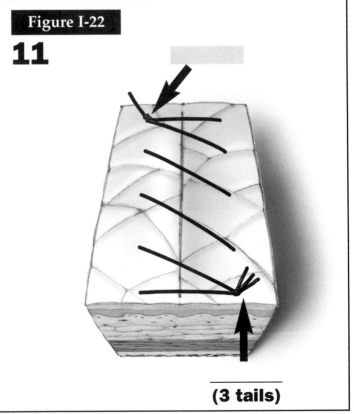

**(3 tails)**

# I. Wound Closure

## f. Running Intracuticular Closure

The running intracuticular closure minimizes penetration of the skin with the needle. This is especially useful in keloid patients where needle holes in the skin may stimulate excessive scar formation. It is also useful in children, since removal is quick and easy compared to all other suture techniques. The needle is placed as a first bite single suture technique approximately 1/2 centimeter to 1 centimeter **from the apex** of the wound **(Figure I-28)**. It is then brought into the ap of the wound in the intracuticular (dermal) layer. Multiple intracuticular bites are then placed opposite each other **(Figures I-29, 30** There is no penetration of the epidermis (skin) except for the first and last bite. If th incision is long (longer than 3 centimeters), then an intermediate bite is used to place a loop, which facilitates suture removal

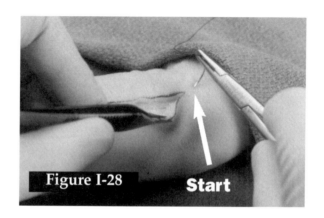

Figure I-28    **Start**

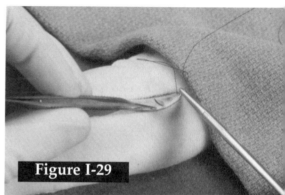

Figure I-29

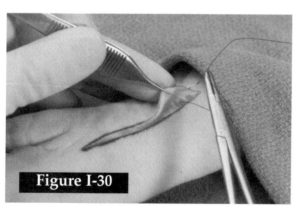

Figure I-30

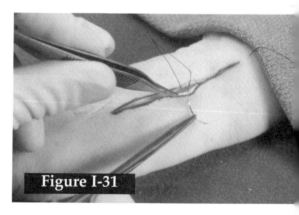

Figure I-31

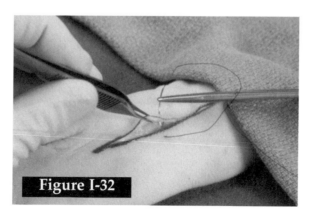

Figure I-32

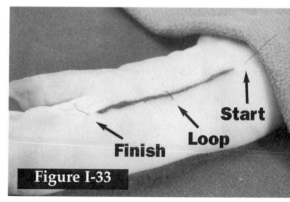

Figure I-33    **Start**  **Loop**  **Finish**

# I. Wound Closure

(**Figures I-31-33**). The needle is drawn back and forth and a loop is brought out every few centimeters (2-3 centimeters) so that the suture can be easily removed without suture fracture (**Figures I-31-33**). This loop is brought out through the skin approximately 1/2 centimeter from the skin edge (**Figure I-33**).

Upon reaching the opposite end of the wound, the needle is placed past the apex of the wound edge and brought out just like at the starting side. Typically, with an intracuticular closure, the wound is reinforced with steri-strips which help reduce tension on the wound. The drawings show the technical details of the running intracuticular closure (**Figure I-34, 1-12**).

## RUNNING INTRACUTICULAR CLOSURE

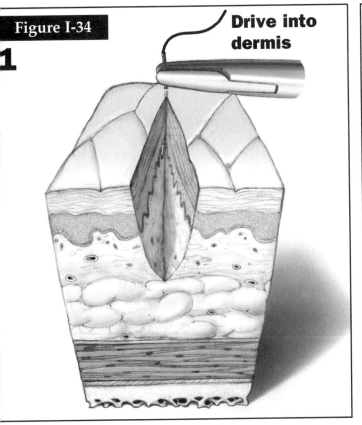

Figure I-34

**1**

**Drive into dermis**

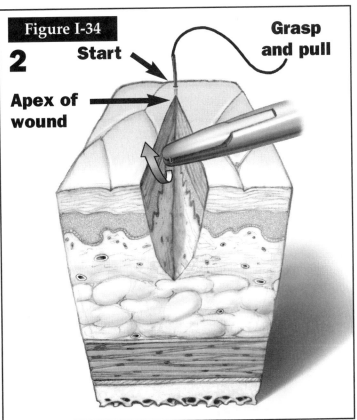

Figure I-34

**2**

**Start**

**Apex of wound**

**Grasp and pull**

# I. Wound Closure

**Figure I-34**

**3**

Drive into dermis on left

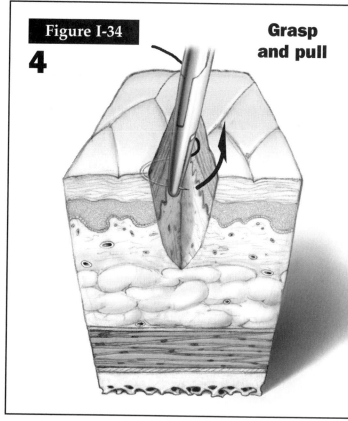

**Figure I-34**

**4**

Grasp and pull

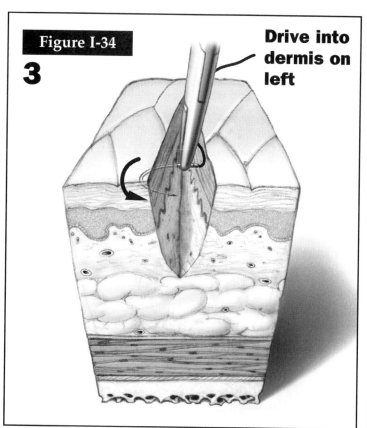

**Figure I-34**

**5**

Start

Apex of wound

Pull

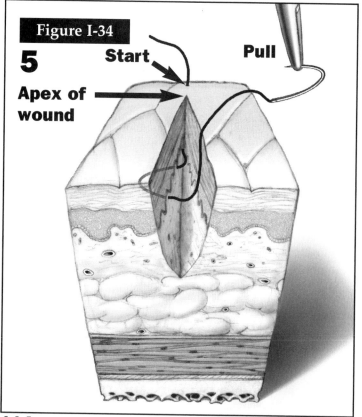

**Figure I-34**

**6**

Drive to start loop

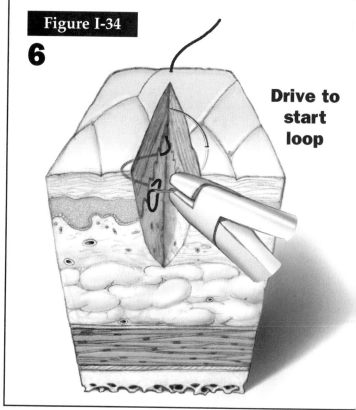

# I. Wound Closure

**Figure I-34**

**7**

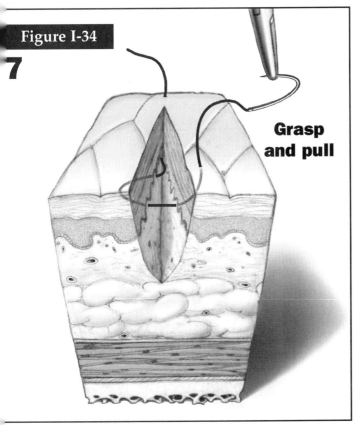

**Grasp and pull**

**Figure I-34**

**8**

**Drive to finish loop**

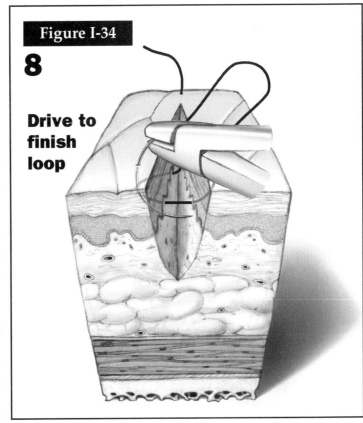

**Figure I-34**

**9**

**Loop**

**Grasp and pull**

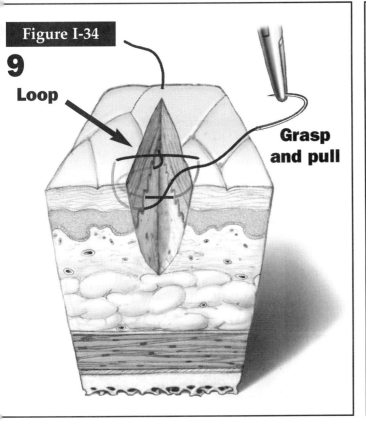

**Figure I-34**

**10**

**Drive into dermis**

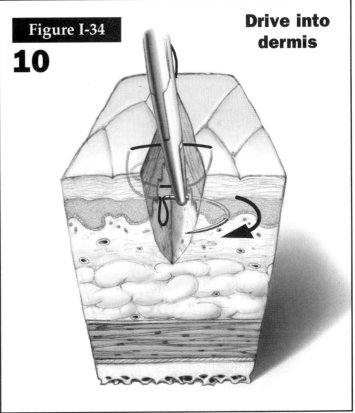

# I. Wound Closure

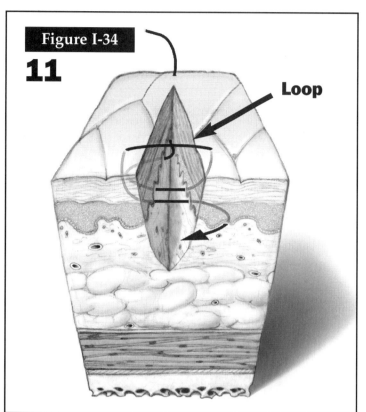

Figure I-34

**11**

Loop

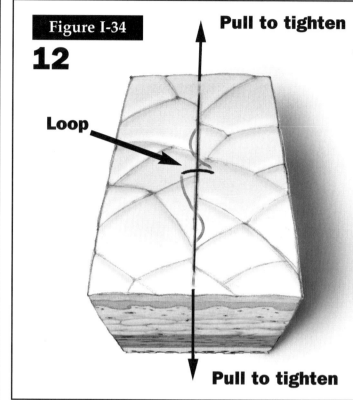

Figure I-34

**12**

**Pull to tighten**

Loop

**Pull to tighten**

# I. Wound Closure

### g. Staples

The staple closure is used for large wounds that are not on the face. Stapling is especially useful for closure of incisions in hair-bearing skin (scalp). The disposable staple gun is held like a normal hand-held stapler **(Figure I-35)**. The wound edge still needs to be everted manually. Each edge is typically picked up with a forceps, everted and precisely lined up **(Figure I-36)**. The surgeon then places the staples to close the wound while the first assistant advances the forceps, everting the edges of the wound. This technique is continued until the entire wound is everted and closed with staples **(Figure I-37)**.

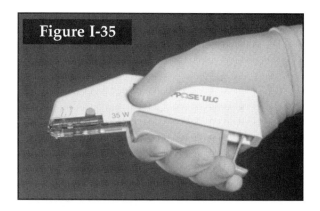

Figure I-35

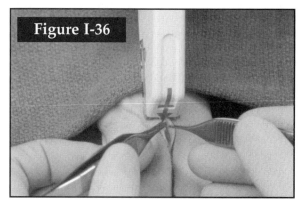

Figure I-36

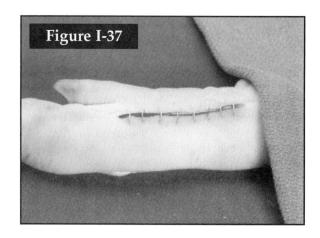

Figure I-37

# I. Wound Closure

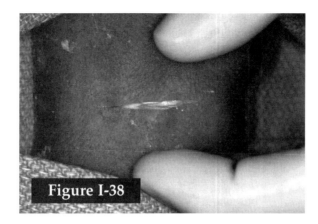

Figure I-38

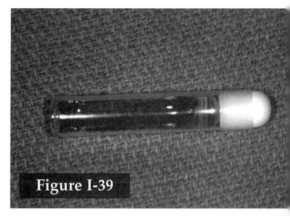

Figure I-39

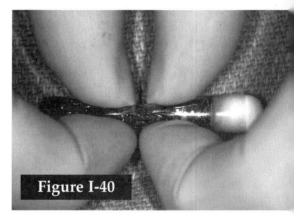

Figure I-40

### h. Skin Adhesive Closure

Low tension wounds can be closed by gluing the skin edges together with a skin adhesive. Everting subcutaneous sutures are used to take all the tension off skin edges after full thickness incisions through the dermis. Thus, low tension wounds are those where the skin edges lie close together without significant tension **(Figure I-38)**. Wounds that are beveled or angled do not close well with a tissue adhesive and require suture skin closure. In those low tension wounds where tissue adhesive can be used, it is quite simple to apply. The liquid skin adhesive is contained in a glass ampule **(Figure I-39)**. The ampule can be crushed by finger pressure **(Figure I-40)**. The applicator tip is moistened with the liquid skin adhesive. The wound edges are held in eversion with a forceps as the skin adhesive is applied along the wound edge and allowed to dry **(Figure I-41)**.

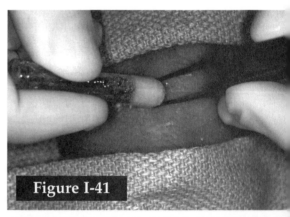

Figure I-41

The adhesive is applied in two or three layers. The wound is kept dry as the skin adhesive seals the wound **(Figure I-42)**. Petroleum-based ointments and similar products dissolve these tissue adhesives, so they should be avoided on postoperative wounds.

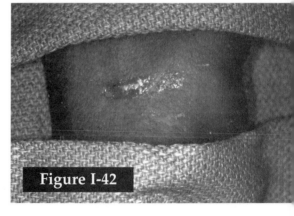

Figure I-42

# I. Wound Closure

**Figure I-43**

**1**

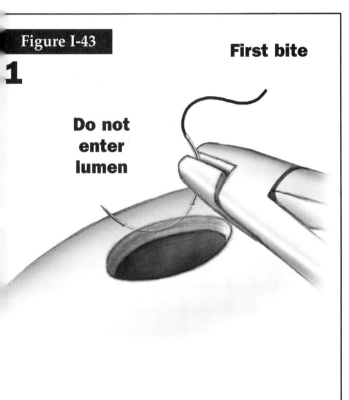

Do not enter lumen

First bite

**Figure I-43**

**2**

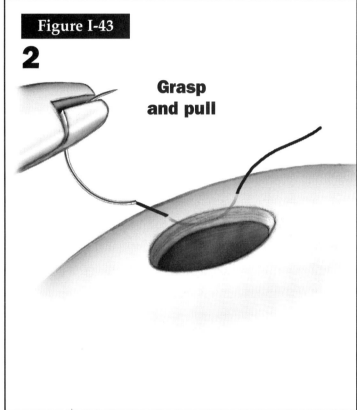

Grasp and pull

**Figure I-43**

**3**

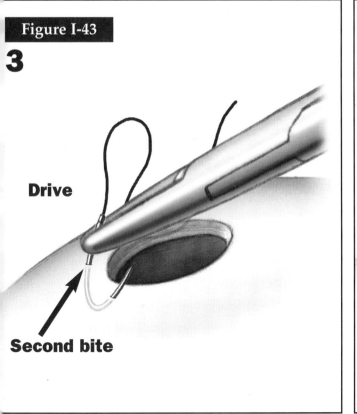

Drive

Second bite

**Figure I-43**

**4**

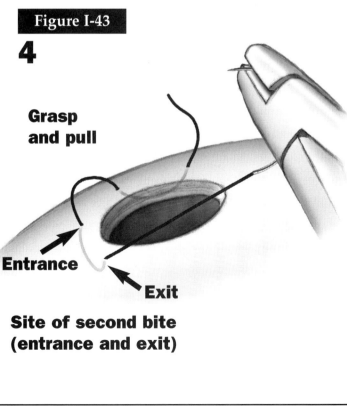

Grasp and pull

Entrance

Exit

Site of second bite (entrance and exit)

# I. Wound Closure

**Figure I-43**

**5**

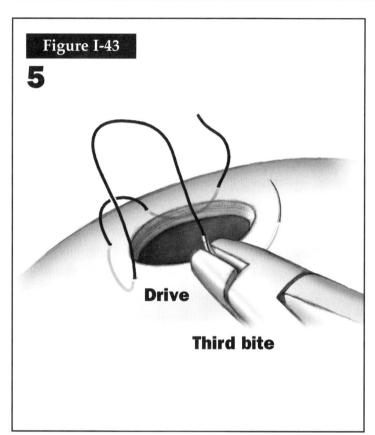

Drive

Third bite

**Figure I-43**

**6**

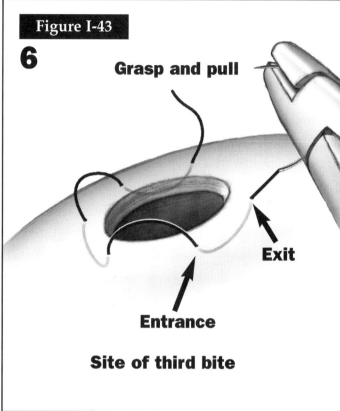

Grasp and pull

Exit

Entrance

Site of third bite

**Figure I-43**

**7**

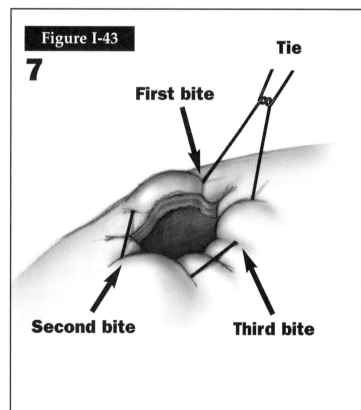

Tie

First bite

Second bite

Third bite

**Figure I-43**

**8**

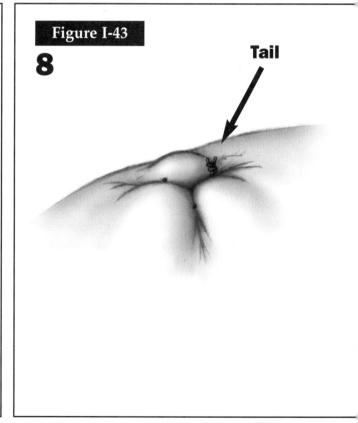

Tail

120

# I. Wound Closure

### i. Purse String Suture

The purse string suture is useful for closing together the edges of a wound where central tissue loss has occurred. Though the edge is irregular at closure the technique may minimize the need for a later local flap or another (revision) surgery. Purse string sutures are especially useful in patients with tissue loss who are not concerned with an optimal cosmetic result. The purse string suture is demonstrated in **Figures I-43, 1-8**.

## 5. Drains

Drains are used to help close the dead space in a wound by removing serum and blood from the deep portions of the wound. Nonsuction drains depend on gravity, while suction drains are attached to a bulb or suction unit **(Figure I-44, 45)**. The drains can be cut to various lengths and fixed to the skin with suture or tape.

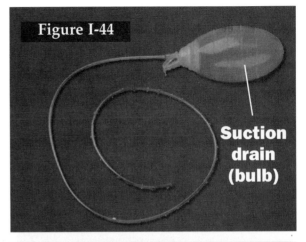

Figure I-44

Suction drain (bulb)

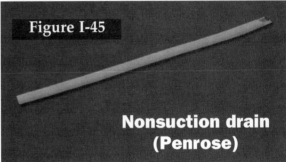

Figure I-45

Nonsuction drain (Penrose)

# J. Skin Flaps

## 1. Introduction

A piece of skin that has been excised (removed) for one reason or another (e.g., it contained a lesion) leaves a hole in the remaining skin. This hole can be closed by a skin flap so that healing can occur by primary intention. Skin flaps optimally close the defect without tension.

Care is taken to stay in the subcutaneous plane during excision of the lesion. Countertraction is helpful during incision and excision. The scissors can be used to undermine as well as cut the deep layers of the soft tissue. The skin incisions themselves should be made with a sharp knife. Incisions should be made perpendicular to the skin edges.

## 2. Fusiform (Elliptical) Excision

Fusiform excision is a simple way to excise skin lesions **(Figure J-1)**. An elliptical incision is made around the lesion, the length of which is 1.5 to 3 times the width of the lesion. If the width-to-length ratio is any closer to 1:1, then the wound will not usually close without puckering at the ends. Once excised, the wound is undermined and closed by the principle of halving **(Figure J-2)**. The drawings **(Figure J-3)** show the technique of the fusiform incision **(Figure J-3A)**, excision **(Figure J-3B)**, undermining **(Figure J-3C)**, and closure **(Figure J-3D)**. The fusiform excision and undermining is a type of advancement flap which allows skin closure without tension.

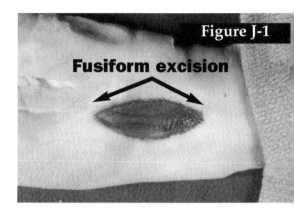

Figure J-1

**Fusiform excision**

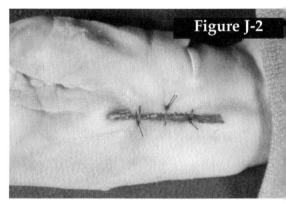

Figure J-2

# J. Skin Flaps

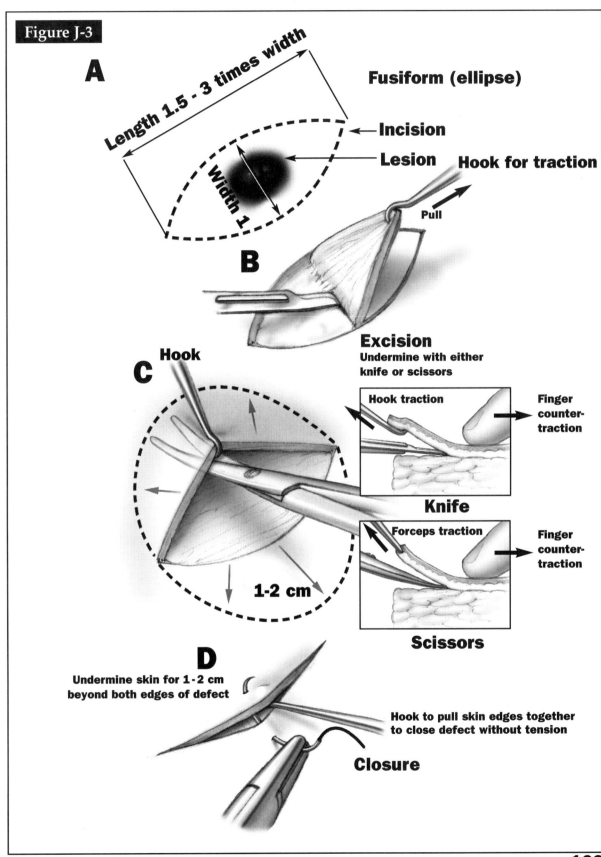

**Figure J-3**

**A**

Length 1.5 - 3 times width

Fusiform (ellipse)

Incision

Lesion

Width 1

**B**

Hook for traction

Pull

Excision
Undermine with either
knife or scissors

Hook traction

Finger counter-traction

**Knife**

**C**

Hook

1-2 cm

Forceps traction

Finger counter-traction

**Scissors**

**D**

Undermine skin for 1-2 cm
beyond both edges of defect

Hook to pull skin edges together
to close defect without tension

**Closure**

# J. Skin Flaps

### 3. Advancement Flap

The advancement flap is rectangular with a 2.5 to 3 length-to-width ratio (**Figure J-4**). The skin defect is in the small shaded square, which is excised. After excision of the lesion, the two sides of the flap are incised and the entire flap is undermined in the layer between the skin and the deeper subcutaneous tissues. The skin adjacent to the long edges of the incision is also undermined for 1-2 centimeters to allow for increased flap mobility and wound closure without tension.

The first suture is placed in the center of the flap and is tied with a hand tie and a surgeon's knot (**Figure J-5**). By keeping constant tension on the sutures, one can prevent tying an "air knot." The suture is cut with a tail to prevent unwinding of the material over time. The corner stitches are placed next, as they are at the other sites of primary tension in this flap design (**Figure J-5**).

Because of the excision, the skin edge is longer than the flap edge (**Figure J-5**). This is closed with the principle of halving. The first suture is placed in the middle of the inferior edge of the flap and in the middle of the corresponding skin (**Figure J-6**). It is tied down and cut. The two halves on either side are still uneven, but less so now. The next suture is placed between the halves of each of these segments. Subsequent sutures then split the difference between previous sutures until enough sutures are placed for an adequate closure (**Figure J-7**). In this way the redundant skin of the lower edge is spread evenly across the entire wound closure and results in a smooth wound edge.

The upper edge is closed in an uneven manner, resulting in a "dog ear," or standing cone, deformity (**Figure J-6**). A standing cone excision is done at this site. First a back cut is made (**Figure J-7**). The standing cone excision is always done away from the flap pedicle to the point of the triangle (**Figure J-8**). Undermining is continued under this standing cone deformity. The skin is moved with a forceps until you can see exactly how much excess skin to trim. The skin is then trimmed and excised appropriately and the flap inset to give a good fit (**Figure J-9**). The flap is then sutured into place and the standing cone deformity is resolved. **Figure J-10** shows the final advancement flap along with the tissue that was excised from the defect. **Figure J-11, A-D** show the technique of correcting a standing cone ("dog ear") deformity. If a flap yields two standing cone ("dog ear") deformities, repair them both.

# J. Skin Flaps

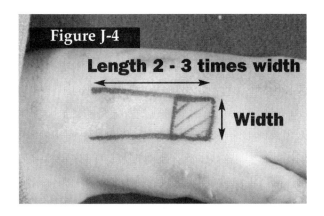

Figure J-4

Length 2 - 3 times width

Width

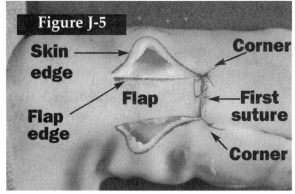

Figure J-5

Skin edge

Corner

Flap

Flap edge

First suture

Corner

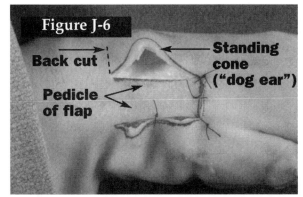

Figure J-6

Back cut

Standing cone ("dog ear")

Pedicle of flap

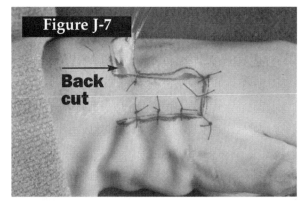

Figure J-7

Back cut

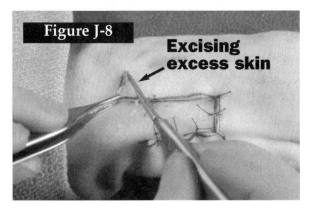

Figure J-8

Excising excess skin

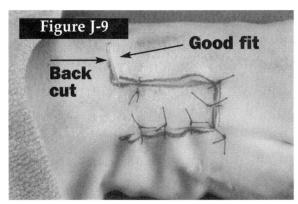

Figure J-9

Back cut

Good fit

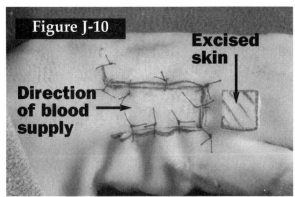

Figure J-10

Excised skin

Direction of blood supply

# J. Skin Flaps

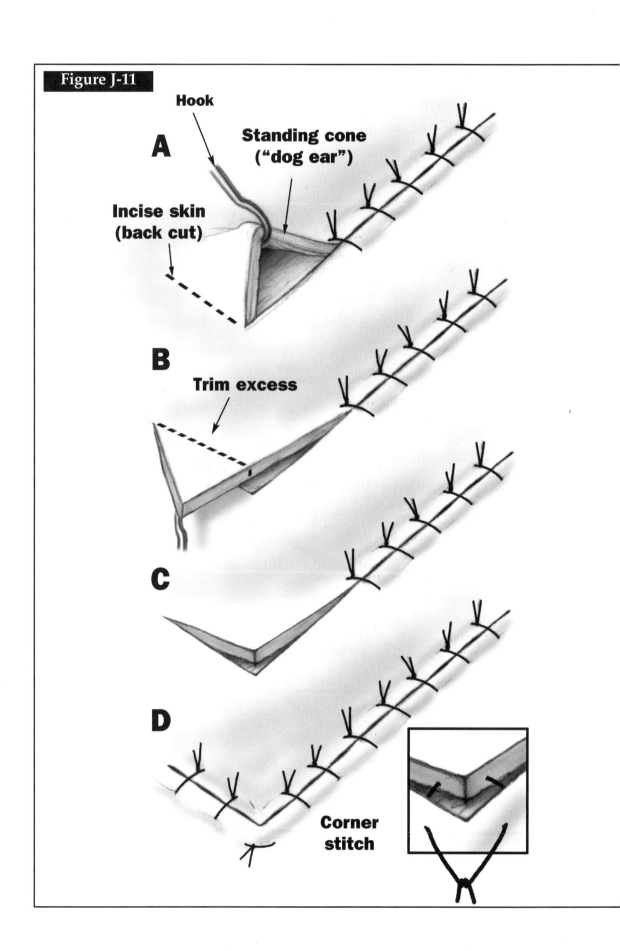

**Figure J-11**

Hook

Standing cone
("dog ear")

**A**

Incise skin
(back cut)

**B**

Trim excess

**C**

**D**

Corner
stitch

# J. Skin Flaps

## 4. Rotation Flap

The rotation flap is utilized to close a triangular defect. The rotation flap follows a smooth curve from the site of the defect. It then gets rotated into place. Typically, the limb of rotation is 2-4 times longer than the axis of the defect it needs to close **(Figure J-12)**. This is a flap with a wide vascular pedicle and is extremely useful in facial reconstruction.

After the lesion is excised, the flap is incised with a knife and broadly undermined. A 1-2 centimeter margin around the skin edges of the defect is also undermined. The point of maximal rotation is also the point of maximal tension in this flap and it is inset first with a suture **(Figure J-13)**. The flap edge is then closed to the longer skin edge with the principle of halving, splitting each side in half for subsequent suture placement. The rotation flap after closure, along with the excised cutaneous defect, is shown in **Figure J-14**.

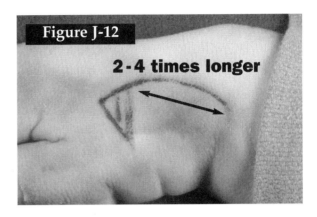

Figure J-12

**2-4 times longer**

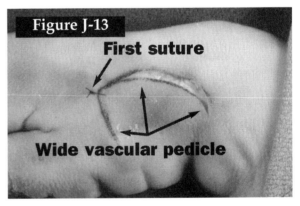

Figure J-13

**First suture**

**Wide vascular pedicle**

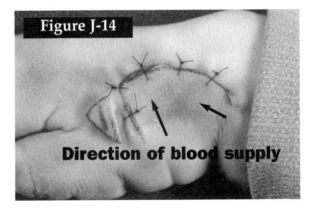

Figure J-14

**Direction of blood supply**

# J. Skin Flaps

## 5. Z-plasty

The Z-plasty is useful in lengthening contracted scars as well as reorienting the direction of scars. In this example the central limb is 3 cm at the start of the incision and would represent the scar to be excised and the axis that we want to lengthen **(Figure J-15)**. The upper flap, A, is stippled to show how it is transposed. This carries the central limb from a horizontal plane to a vertical plane **(Figures J-15-17)**. The limbs are the same length and both come off at the same angle from the central limb. The angle varies anywhere between 30 and 60°. The greater the angle, the greater the gain in wound length. Any sharper angle results in risk of necrosis in the tip of the flap, while any broader angle results in a difficult rotation. Both triangular flaps rotate opposite each other. Broad undermining is done under both flaps, as well as under the entire incised region, to allow ease of flap elevation and rotation. Each flap is then grasped with a forceps and transposed across so that the central limb totally reorients by 90° in this example **(Figure J-16)**. The width of the defect increased from 3-4 centimeters, demonstrating the lengthening effect of a Z-plasty **(Figure J-17)**. The corner stitches are placed into each flap first to transpose them. Always remember to transpose the Z-plasty. If it is closed as it was initially incised, it will have no effect.

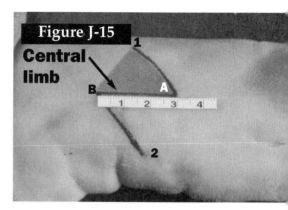

**Figure J-15**

**Central limb**

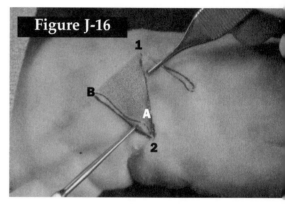

**Figure J-16**

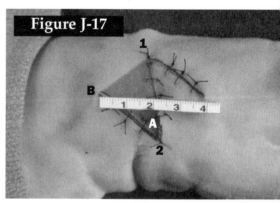

**Figure J-17**

# Quiz

Fill in the shaded blanks! See page 126, Figure J-11 for the correct answers.

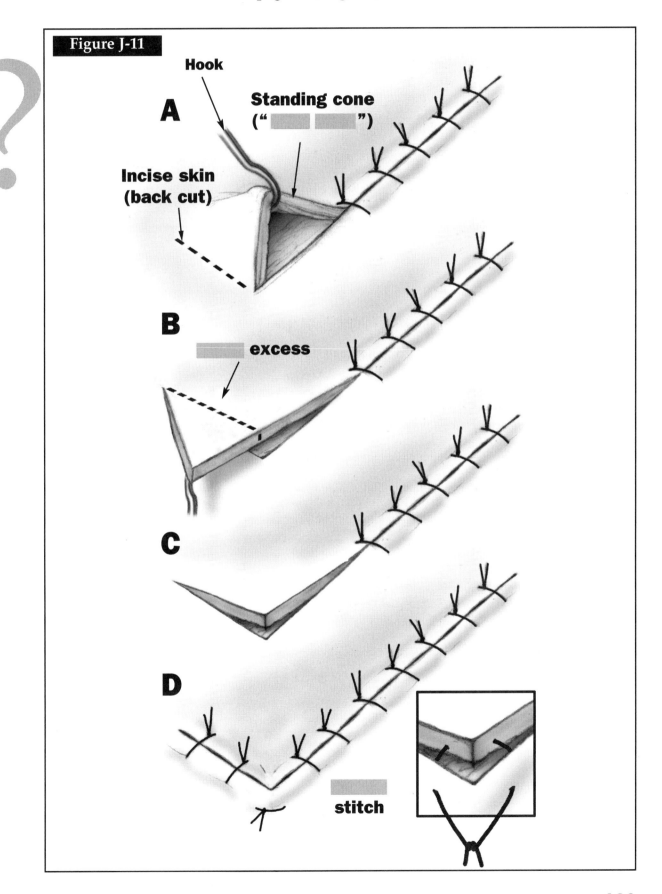

**Figure J-11**

**A** Hook

Standing cone
("▨▨▨ ▨▨▨▨")

Incise skin
(back cut)

**B** ▨▨▨▨ excess

**C**

**D** ▨▨▨▨ stitch

# K. Postoperative Wound Care

## 1. Local Wound Care

In general it is best to keep the wound dry during healing. Avoid allowing excessive moisture in and around the wound. It may be helpful for the patient to clean the wound with alcohol or hydrogen peroxide to remove blood debris and "crusts" of dried blood. Antibiotic ointment may be placed on the sutures two or three times a day to keep them from getting crusted.

When bathing, it may be necessary to cover the wound with a piece of plastic. On postoperative visits, reexamine the wound, especially if the patient complains of pain or tenderness. Observe the wound for swelling, redness (**erythema**), tenderness to palpation, and drainage from the wound. The patient may also experience fear. If any of these findings occur, it may be necessary to reopen the wound to make sure that an abscess is not forming.

## 2. Steri-Strips

Steri-strips are used to close very low tension wounds. They help keep the wound edges together (**Figures K-1-5**). Steri-strips can also be useful to help keep the wound covered and its edges together even after skin sutures have been placed. They can be especially helpful after intracuticular closures.

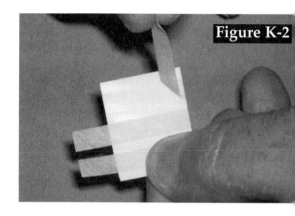
Figure K-2

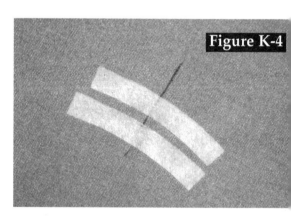
Figure K-3

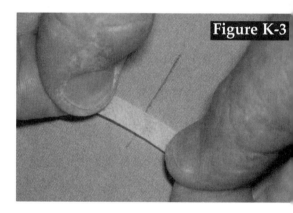
Figure K-4

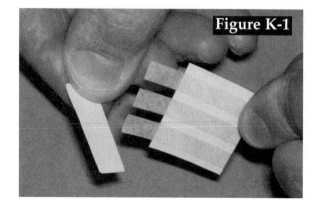
Figure K-1

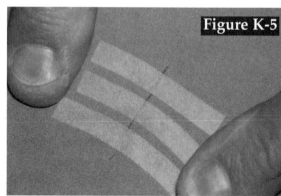
Figure K-5

# K. Postoperative Wound Care

## 3. Suture Removal

The time for suture removal depends upon the location of the wound, but in the facial region, it usually ranges from the fifth to the seventh postoperative day. It is usually best to pick up the knotted end of the suture with fine forceps. A suture-removal scissors is then applied to cut the suture and remove it as atraumatically as possible. On occasion, it may be necessary, after sutures have been removed, to then apply steri-strips to help support the wound, especially if removal is on or about the fifth day.

### a. Simple Suture Removal

Note how in **Figure K-6,** the knotted end is grasped with the pickup forceps, and the distal end is cut adjacent to the skin. **Figure K-7** demonstrates the removal of the simple suture so that the edge of the suture is not dragged through the wound. Be sure **not to cut** the sutures in 2 spots; otherwise, you have nothing to pull the suture through the wound. You do not want to leave a permanent suture in the wound.

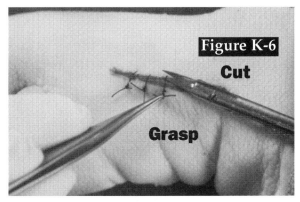

Figure K-6
Cut
Grasp

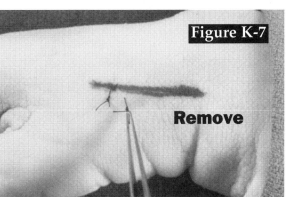

Figure K-7
Remove

# K. Postoperative Wound Care

**b. Vertical Mattress Suture Removal**
Grasp the knotted end with a fine forceps and cut the looped end with the fine suture scissors **(Figure K-8)**. **Figure K-9** demonstrates the removal of the suture.

**c. Horizontal Mattress Suture Removal**
Grasp the knotted end and cut the suture on the opposite side to remove the suture atraumatically **(Figures K-10,11)**.

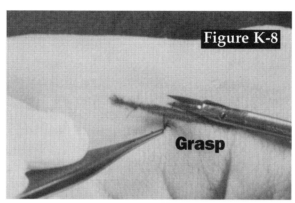

Figure K-8 · Grasp

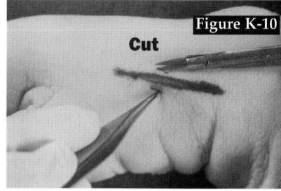

Figure K-10 · Cut

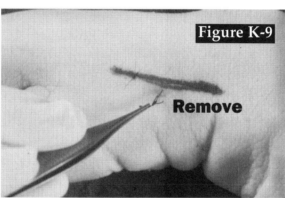

Figure K-9 · Remove

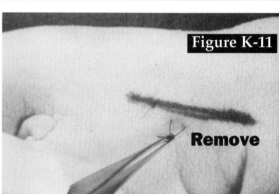

Figure K-11 · Remove

# K. Postoperative Wound Care

**d. Simple Running Suture ("Baseball Stitch") Removal**

Grasp one knotted end and use the suture scissors to cut the looped end **(Figure K-12)**. Continue cutting the looped ends **(Figure K-13)**. Once you reach the other knotted end at the extreme end of the wound, remove each loop just as if you were removing simple sutures **(Figure K-14)**.

**e. Running-lock Suture Removal**

Again, start at one end, grasping the knot, and use a fine suture scissors to cut the loop **(Figure K-15)**. Proceed down the wound, cutting the locked loops as you continue down to the end of the suture line **(Figure K-16)**. Then remove each suture individually as if you were removing a simple suture **(Figure K-17)**.

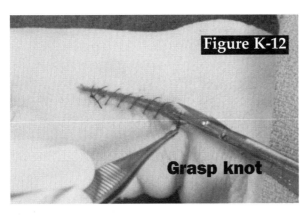

Figure K-12

Grasp knot

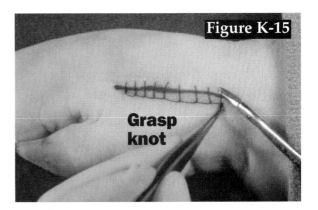

Figure K-15

Grasp knot

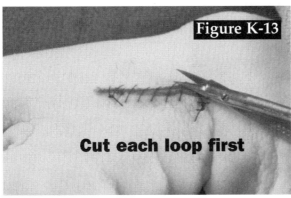

Figure K-13

Cut each loop first

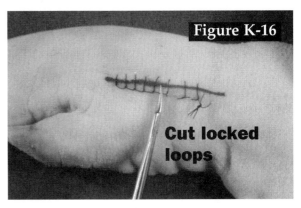

Figure K-16

Cut locked loops

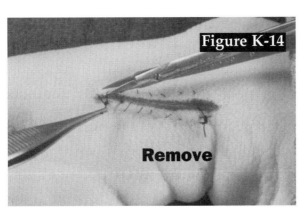

Figure K-14

Remove

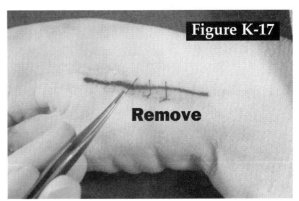

Figure K-17

Remove

# K. Postoperative Wound Care

**f. Running Intracuticular Suture Removal**
Cut the suture loop in the midportion of the wound **(Figure K-18)**. Extract the suture on the left side of the wound with forceps **(Figure K-19)**. Then extract the suture on the right side of the wound with forceps **(Figure K-20)**.

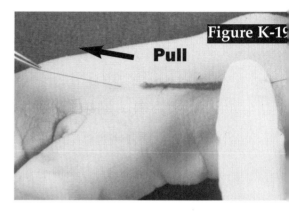

Figure K-19

Pull

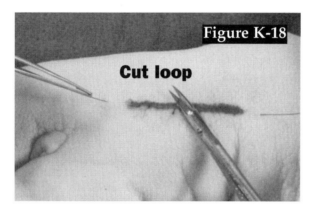

Figure K-18

Cut loop

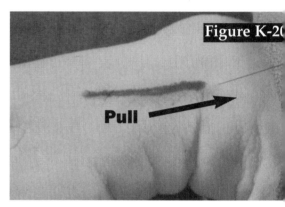

Figure K-20

Pull

# K. Postoperative Wound Care

## 4. Staple Removal

Pick up the staple removal instrument and approach the wound along its long axis **(Figure K-21)**. Then engage the staple removal instrument beneath the staple **(Figure K-22).** Close the staple removal instrument and extract the staple **(Figure K-23)**. Continue until all the staples are removed **(Figure K-24)**. On occasion, it may be necessary to use steri-strips to help keep small portions of the wound which have **dehisced** (come apart) in proper position.

## 5. Drain Removal

Most drains are sutured in place with a simple suture. All that is necessary is to cut the suture with the suture scissors. Grasp the knotted end with the forceps and remove the suture. Once the suture is removed the drain will be free to be shortened, cut, or completely extracted. Suction drains should be removed from suction by deflating the bulb prior to removal.

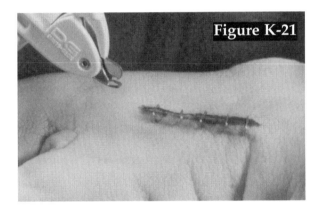

Figure K-21

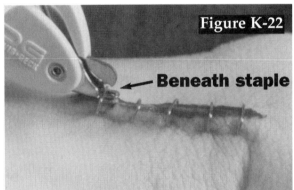

Figure K-22

Beneath staple

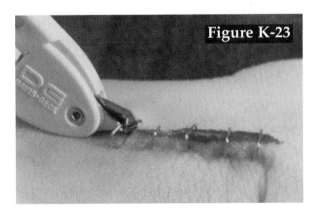

Figure K-23

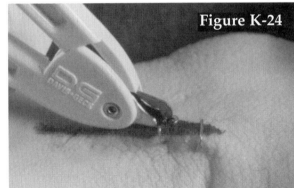

Figure K-24

# L. Quiz Questions

How about a quick quiz? If you cannot answer a question, read further. The answers are provided on page 145. No peeking! Circle the best choice before checking the answers.

1. An anesthesiologist is:
   a. a surgeon
   b. a physician specializing in administration of anesthetics
   c. a physician specializing in the lung
   d. a physician specializing in the gastrointestinal tract
   e. none of the above

2. Bacteremia
   a. an infection
   b. bacteria in the gastrointestinal tract
   c. the presence of bacteria in the blood
   d. the presence of bacteria in the urine
   e. none of the above

3. Cardiopulmonary
   a. pertaining to the heart and lungs
   b. pertaining to the heart
   c. pertaining to the lungs
   d. pertaining to the kidney
   e. all of the above

4. Cellulitis
   a. inflammation of cells
   b. inflammation of fat
   c. inflammation of the brain
   d. inflammation of muscle
   e. none of the above

5. Cicatrix
   a. a scar
   b. a wound
   c. a part of the kidney
   d. a part of bone
   e. all of the above

6. Collagen
   a. a blood-borne substance
   b. substance present in neurologic tissue
   c. the protein substance of connective tissues
   d. the mineralized matrix of bone
   e. all of the above

7. Debridement
   a. the process of making an incision
   b. the removal of foreign material or dead tissue
   c. the laying down of bone by osteoblasts
   d. the process of obtaining hemostasis
   e. none of the above

8. Dehiscence
   a. the removal of foreign material
   b. the act of removing diseased tissue
   c. the separation of the layers of a surgical wound
   d. the falling apart of a wound
   e. both c and d

9. Devitalized
   a. to deprive of vitality or of life
   b. the removal of internal organs
   c. the death of tissue
   d. all of the above
   e. a and c

10. Electrolyte
    a. sodium
    b. chloride
    c. substance that dissociates-associates into ions when in solution
    d. potassium
    e. all of the above

11. "Endocrine" means:
    a. pertaining to internal secretion of a hormonal nature
    b. pertaining to blood-borne bacteria
    c. pertaining to the elements of blood
    d. pertaining to neurologic tissue
    e. none of the above

12. "Enzyme" means:
    a. a substance that is changed during a chemical reaction
    b. a protein molecule that participates in a chemical reaction by speeding the chemical reaction
    c. a carbohydrate moiety that speeds chemical reactions
    d. none of the above
    e. all of the above

13. Epinephrine is:
    a. a primary constituent of bone
    b. a drug used to open clogged blood vessels
    c. a vasoconstrictive agent that causes blood vessels to narrow or shrink down
    d. none of the above
    e. all of the above

14. "Erythematous" means:
    a. whiteness of the skin
    b. redness of the skin
    c. loss of vascular supply to the skin
    d. dullness of the skin
    e. loss of tissue oxygenation

# L. Quiz Questions

15. Fibroblasts are:
    a. a red blood cell
    b. a kidney cell
    c. a cardiac muscle cell
    d. a smooth muscle cell
    e. a connective-tissue cell producing collagen

16. Gangrene is:
    a. loss of kidney function
    b. loss of the ability of the lungs to work adequately
    c. death of tissue secondary to trauma
    d. death of tissue due to a loss of vascular supply followed by infection
    e. none of the above

17. The formation in wounds of fleshy masses, which include a large amount of new blood vessels, during the healing process is:
    a. angiogenesis
    b. scar
    c. gangrene
    d. granulation tissue
    e. none of the above

18. A collection of blood in an organ or tissue due to a break in the wall of the blood vessel is:
    a. a hematoma
    b. the swollen space that contains blood
    c. an abscess
    d. all of the above
    e. a and b

19. The interruption of the flow of blood through any vessel to any anatomical area is known as:
    a. cellulitis
    b. dehiscence
    c. erythema
    d. keloid
    e. hemostasis

20. HIV stands for:
    a. the human immunodeficiency virus
    b. the virus that causes AIDS (acquired immunodeficiency syndrome)
    c. hepatic immunodeficiency virus
    d. all of the above
    e. a and b

21. The overgrowth of scar tissue is known as:
    a. osteogenesis scar
    b. geographic scar
    c. tumor-like scar
    d. devitalization cicatrix
    e. hypertrophic scar

22. The body system that protects against infection and infectious disease is known as:
    a. the endocrine system
    b. the musculoskeletal system
    c. the pulmonary system
    d. the collagen system
    e. none of the above

23. The body's protective response caused by injury or destruction of tissue is known as:
    a. inflammation
    b. angiogenesis
    c. embryogenesis
    d. reflex
    e. symptomatology

24. Intubation is:
    a. the placement of a tube into a body canal or hollow organ
    b. the placement of a tube into the trachea
    c. the placement of a tube into the stomach
    d. all of the above
    e. none of the above

25. Keloids are:
    a. broken bones
    b. renal cells
    c. the end result of all scarring
    d. enlarged scar due to formation of excessive amounts of collagen
    e. enlarged scar due to formation of excessive amounts of cartilage

26. Lymphocytes are:
    a. red blood cells found in the blood, lymph, and lymphoid tissues
    b. white blood cells found in the blood, lymph, and lymphoid tissues
    c. tumor cells
    d. cells which reproduce in an uncontrolled manner by sexual reproduction
    e. none of the above

27. The sum of all the physical and chemical processes by which living organisms maintain their function and survive is known as:
    a. metaphysical functions
    b. holistic functions
    c. metabolic functions
    d. biochemical functions
    e. anabolic functions

28. A nurse trained in the administration of anesthetics is known as:
    a. an anesthesiologist
    b. a somnologist
    c. a nurse anesthetist
    d. an oncologist
    e. none of the above

29. The branch of medicine which studies basic elements of disease, especially changes in the body caused by disease, is:
    a. ophthalmology
    b. biochemistry
    c. oncology
    d. otorhinolaryngology
    e. pathology

30. "Perioperative" pertains to:
    a. the time period just before surgery
    b. the time period from the time of surgery to the time of discharge from the hospital
    c. the time period from one day prior to one day post-surgery
    d. two of the above
    e. all of the above

31. The time period occurring after a surgical operation is known as:
    a. postoperative
    b. perioperative
    c. operative
    d. two of the above
    e. all of the above

32. A seroma is also known as:
    a. a hematoma
    b. a chyloma
    c. a collection of serum in the tissues
    d. a serous cell tumor
    e. two of the above

33. Serum is:
    a. a body fluid consisting of vascular fluid devoid of white blood cells
    b. a body fluid consisting of vascular fluid devoid of white blood cells and platelets
    c. a body fluid consisting of vascular fluid devoid of red blood cells
    d. a body fluid consisting of vascular fluid devoid of platelets
    e. none of the above

34. The branch of medicine which treats disease, injuries, and deformities by operation is:
    a. psychiatry
    b. internal medicine
    c. obstetrics
    d. pediatrics
    e. surgery

35. The term vasoconstrictive describes:
    a. a diminished caliber of blood vessels
    b. the loss of fatty tissues
    c. to narrow or shrink down blood vessels
    d. all of the above
    e. a and c

36. Viscera describes:
    a. the internal organs located inside the body cavity
    b. the renal system
    c. the hematopoietic system
    d. the musculoskeletal system
    e. the neurologic system

37. Tissue layers include:
    a. skin
    b. subcutaneous tissue
    c. fascia
    d. periosteum
    e. all of the above

38. The removal of damaged and dead tissue in a wound occurs during:
    a. the inflammation stage
    b. the proliferation of scar formation stage
    c. the scar maturation stage
    d. all of the above
    e. none of the above

39. Scar maturation:
    a. occurs immediately following the inflammatory stage
    b. occurs on days 5-14 and consists of the initiation of production of collagen fibers
    d. is not a distinct phase of wounding
    e. has a variable duration depending upon the specific type of tissues that are wounded

# L. Quiz Questions

40. The epidermis is part of the:
    a. subcutaneous tissue
    b. muscle
    c. periosteum
    d. skin
    e. bone

41. Periosteum covers bone like fascia covers:
    a. skin
    b. fat
    c. muscle
    d. lung
    e. bladder

42. Subcutaneous tissue includes:
    a. skin
    b. connective tissue
    c. muscle
    d. fat
    e. b and d

43. Scar maturation occurs:
    a. as the last stage of tissue repair
    b. after all wounding including tattoos
    c. after the inflammatory stage
    d. all of the above
    e. none of the above

44. The only stage in which collagen fibers do not play a major role is:
    a. scar maturation
    b. proliferation and scar formation
    c. inflammation
    d. all of the above
    e. none of the above

45. Wound closure using sutures is termed:
    a. closure by primary intention
    b. closure by secondary intention
    c. granulation
    d. hemostasis
    e. none of the above

46. If during the course of an operation in which an initially clean wound was made and the pharyngeal cavity was entered, the wound is now:
    a. still a clean wound
    b. a contaminated wound
    c. a clean, contaminated wound
    d. an infected wound
    e. none of the above

47. "Dirty" wounds are:
    a. those which occur during sexual activity
    b. an already contaminated wound, for example, an abscess
    c. a wound which is initially clean but then the gastrointestinal tract is entered
    d. b and c

48. Factors which affect wound healing include:
    a. age
    b. steroids
    c. anti-neoplastic drugs
    d. weight
    e. all of the above

49. Factors which affect blood supply, and therefore wound healing, include:
    a. poor circulation secondary to cardiac dysfunction
    b. diabetes
    c. various vascular illnesses
    d. all of the above
    e. none of the above

50. Factors which affect wound healing include:
    a. chronic illness
    b. radiation therapy
    c. nutrition
    d. a and c
    e. all of the above

51. Complications seen in wound healing include:
    a. cellulitis
    b. scar maturation
    c. inflammation
    d. healing by tertiary intention
    e. none of the above

52. After primary closure about 95 percent of wound strength is reached by:
    a. six days
    b. six months
    c. six weeks
    d. four weeks
    e. fourteen days

53. Clean, contaminated wounds would include initially clean wounds which were then contaminated by:
    a. entrance into the pharyngeal cavity
    b. entrance into the genitourinary cavity
    c. entrance into the heart
    d. a and b
    e. none of the above

54. Contaminated wounds are also known as infected wounds. They are made through an already infected area where gross contamination by bacteria and/or other microorganisms are already present. We are giving you the answer so that you will not embarrass the authors by ever forgetting the definition of contaminated or infected wounds.

55. The method of wound closure during which the wound is only allowed to granulate closed is called:
    a. healing by primary intention
    b. healing by secondary intention
    c. healing by tertiary intention
    d. healing by quaternary intention
    e. none of the above

56. Hematomas usually result from:
    a. dehiscence of the wound
    b. cellulitis
    c. failure to obtain hemostasis at surgery
    d. a and b
    e. none of the above

57. Relaxed skin tension lines are:
    a. not important during surgery
    b. important for planning incisions
    c. the lines of minimal intention of the skin
    d. all of the above
    e. b and c

58. Areas of the wound that have not been adequately closed are called:
    a. dehiscences
    b. hematomas
    c. dead spaces
    d. seromas
    e. horrenudomas

59. Choice of suture material:
    a. is irrelevant
    b. depends upon the tissues and area of the body where the wound is to be closed
    c. is usually left up to the scrub nurse
    d. is whatever the hospital gives you
    e. all of the above

60. Basic principles in surgery include:
    a. relaxed skin tension lines
    b. incision planning
    c. tissue moisture
    d. hemostasis
    e. all of the above

61. Local anesthetics:
    a. prevent the sensation of pain
    b. work by blocking nerve conduction
    c. can be administered topically
    d. all of the above
    e. a and c

62. Which of the following is true?
    a. lidocaine's onset is immediate
    b. bupivacaine has a shorter duration than lidocaine
    c. procaine has a longer duration than bupivacaine
    d. the onset of action of all three is greater than five minutes
    e. all of the above

63. Which of the following is true?
    a. cocaine is a topical anesthetic
    b. lidocaine is both a topical and injectable anesthetic
    c. bupivacaine is primarily used as a vasoconstrictive agent
    d. a and b
    e. none of the above

64. The gauge of a needle refers to:
    a. its length
    b. the needle bore
    c. the needle diameter
    d. b and c
    e. none of the above

65. A wound under excessive postoperative stress can be caused by:
    a. exercise
    b. is not important in an adequately closed wound
    c. never contributes to seroma formation
    d. none of the above
    e. all of the above

66. Local anesthetics:
    a. are often used in combination with vaso-constrictive agents
    b. can reduce perioperative and postoperative pain
    c. can reduce the incidences of nausea and vomiting often associated with general anesthetics
    d. can facilitate earlier discharge from the hospital
    e. all of the above

67. Patients who are not good candidates for local anesthetics include:
    a. patients with a language barrier
    b. calm, cooperative patients
    c. anxious adults
    d. severely emotionally disturbed patients
    e. a, c and d

68. By Kern's rule, a 2% lidocaine solution has:
    a. 10 mg per cc
    b. 20 mg per cc
    c. 40 mg per cc
    d. 80 mg per cc
    e. none of the above

69. The reason a test dose is given when injecting local anesthetics is:
    a. since medical students are tortured so much, it is felt that everyone needs to be tested as much as possible
    b. to see if the drug will work
    c. to make sure no adverse reactions occur
    d. none of the above
    e. all of the above

70. Which of the following is true?
    a. the #10 blade is held at a 45-degree angle
    b. the #10 blade is held like a steak knife
    c. the #10 blade is held like a pencil
    d. the # 15 blade is held at a 30-degree angle
    e. a and c

71. The #10 blade is held at:
    a. a 30° angle
    b. like a steak knife
    c. at a 45° angle
    d. a and b
    e. b and c

72. The #15 blade is:
    a. larger than a #10 blade
    b. smaller than a #10 blade
    c. held at a 30° angle
    d. held like a steak knife
    e. not typically used for facial surgery

73. Tissue scissors:
    a. are also known as dissection scissors or undermining scissors
    b. are used to elevate or separate tissues
    c. usually have tips that are blunted
    d. a and c
    e. all of the above

74. Needle holders come in several varieties, including:
    a. those with jaws with teeth
    b. those used for injection
    c. those without teeth
    d. a and c
    e. all of the above

75. The hemostat:
    a. can be either straight or curved
    b. can be used to dissect
    c. can be used as a needle holder
    d. should be held with the thumb and third finger in the ring holes
    e. a and b

76. A tail is left on a suture:
    a. for cosmetic purposes
    b. to give something that can be grasped to facilitate removal
    c. to prevent knot slippage, loosening, and undoing of the suture
    d. all of the above
    e. b and c

77. Electrocautery:
    a. is used for hemostasis
    b. comes in monopolar and bipolar forms
    c. works by using electrical current to coagulate blood vessels
    d. all of the above
    e. b and c

# L. Quiz Questions

78. Monopolar cautery:
    a. generates less heat than bipolar
    b. can be used to cut tissues
    c. is usually used to cut skin
    d. transmits less heat to the surrounding tissue than bipolar cautery
    e. all of the above

79. A wound closure:
    a. can be facilitated by undermining of the skin surrounding the wound
    b. is rarely necessary
    c. should be done by closing anatomic layers
    d. a and c
    e. none of the above

80. A 6-0 suture is:
    a. larger diameter than a 4-0
    b. smaller diameter than a 4-0
    c. is too small for skin closure
    d. b and c
    e. none of the above

81. In children or noncompliant adults:
    a. absorbable suture is a good choice
    b. local anesthesia is a poor choice
    c. suture removal can be difficult in the case of children because of their failure to understand the need for it and their inherent fear of pain, and in the case of noncompliant adults because they may not show up for their follow-up appointment
    d. a and c
    e. all of the above

82. The two-hand tie:
    a. gives the best knot security
    b. is rarely used in surgery
    c. is not a tremendously useful tie
    d. b and c
    e. none of the above

83. In regard to suction devices:
    a. continuous suctions have a hole that can be plugged or unplugged
    b. intermittent suctions have a side port hole that should never be plugged
    c. suctions come in various types, including continuous suctions and intermittent suctions
    d. suctions are used to remove fluids from the field but should not be used to remove blood from the field due to risk of clotting off the suction
    e. on a continuous suction, when a side port hole is unplugged, the suction is turned off

84. The surgeon's knot:
    a. is the same as a square knot
    b. has two loops in the first throw
    c. is useful because the first throw with the two loops tends to stay in place better than the square knot
    d. b and c
    e. none of the above

85. Skin flaps can be used to:
    a. provide tissue coverage in wounds that have a tissue defect
    b. improve cosmetic results
    c. slow wound healing to an appropriate speed
    d. achieve homeostasis
    e. a and b

86. The rotation flap:
    a. is appropriate for closing a circular defect
    b. is appropriate for closing a square defect
    c. is used to provide skin coverage when the is skin loss
    d. is appropriate for closing a triangular defect
    e. c and d

87. The Z-plasty:
    a. is useful in shortening wounds
    b. is useful in reorienting the direction of scar
    c. provides no improvement in cosmesis ever
    d. is a free flap
    e. is only used for closing square defects

88. Various types of skin flaps include:
    a. the advancement flap
    b. the rotation flap
    c. the Dennis Rodman tattoo flap
    d. a and b
    e. none of the above

89. The Z-plasty, the rotation flap, and the advancement flap are all types of:
    a. local skin flaps
    b. complications of wound healing
    c. hypertrophic scars
    d. microvascular free flaps
    e. none of the above

90. The surgeon's knot:
    a. can be done as an instrument tie
    b. can be done as a two-hand tie
    c. can be done only by the surgeon
    d. b and c
    e. a and b

# M. Glossary of Terms

anesthesiologist . . . .a physician specializing in administration of anesthetics

antineoplastic . . . . .inhibiting or preventing the development of cancer

bacteremia . . . . . . . .the presence of bacteria in the blood

bevel . . . . . . . . . . . .a slanting edge

cardiopulmonary . . .pertaining to the heart and lungs

cellulitis . . . . . . . . . .inflammation of the subcutaneous tissues

cicatrix . . . . . . . . . . .a scar; the new tissue formed in the healing of a wound

collagen . . . . . . . . . .the protein substance of connective tissues; part of scar formation in wound healing

debridement . . . . . . .the removal of foreign material

dehiscence . . . . . . . .separation of the layers of a surgical wound; the falling apart of the wound

devitalized . . . . . . . .to deprive of vitality or of life; the death of tissue

electrocardiogram . . .(ECG) a graphic tracing of the electrical activity of the heart muscle

electrolyte . . . . . . . . .a substance that dissociates into ions when in solution and is capable of conducting electricity; important elements in tissue fluids, like sodium, chloride, and potassium

endocrine . . . . . . . . .pertaining to internal secretions; hormonal; related to endocrine glands like thyroid, adrenal, pituitary, pancreas and thymus

enzyme . . . . . . . . . .a protein molecule that speeds chemical reactions of other substances without being altered or destroyed itself

epinephrine . . . . . . . .a vasoconstrictive agent that causes blood vessels to narrow or shrink down

erythematous . . . . . .redness of the skin

fibroblast . . . . . . . . .a connective tissue cell

gangrene . . . . . . . . .death of tissue due to a loss of vascular supply followed by infection

granulation tissue . .the formation of flesh masses, including new blood vessels, which appear in the wound during the healing process

hematoma . . . . . . . .a collection of blood in an organ or tissue due to a break in the wall of a blood vessel; the swollen space that contains blood

# M. Glossary of Terms

**hemostasis** . . . . . . . . .interruption of the flow of blood through any vessel or to any anatomical area

**HIV** . . . . . . . . . . . .human immunodeficiency virus; the virus that causes AIDS (acquired immuno-deficiency syndrome)

**hypertrophic scars** . .hypertrophy; overgrowth and widening of scar tissue

**immune** . . . . . . . . . .the body's protective response caused by injury or destruction of tissues

**intubation** . . . . . . . .placement of a tube into a body canal or hollow organ, as into the trachea or stomach

**keloids** . . . . . . . . . . .enlarged scars that extend beyond the limits of the original incision due to formation of excessive amounts of collagen

**leukocytes** . . . . . . . .white blood cells

**lymphocytes** . . . . . .white blood cells found in the blood, lymph, and lymphoid tissues

**metabolic** . . . . . . . . .all chemical changes that occur in living tissue

**metabolism** . . . . . . . .the sum of all the physical and chemical processes by which living organisms maintain their function and survive

**necrosis** . . . . . . . . . .tissue death

**nurse anesthetist** . . .a nurse (male or female) trained in the administration of anesthetics

**oxygen saturation** . . .the percent of oxygen bound to available hemoglobin

**pathology** . . . . . . . .that branch of medicine which studies basic elements of disease, especially changes in the body caused by disease

**perioperative** . . . . . .pertaining to the time period from the time of surgery to the time of discharge from the hospital

**postoperative** . . . . . .time period occurring after a surgical operation

**radiation therapy** . . . . . . .treatment of cancers and other conditions with x-rays or any other appropriate rays

**seroma** . . . . . . . . . . .a collection of serum in the tissues

**serum** . . . . . . . . . . . .body fluid, vascular fluid devoid of red blood cells

**sterile** . . . . . . . . . . . .the state of being aseptic or free of all microorganisms or spores

**surgery** . . . . . . . . . . .that branch of medicine which treats diseases, injuries and deformities by manual or operative methods

**vasoconstrictive** . . . .characterized by a decrease in the diameter of a blood vessel; to narrow or shrink down blood vessels

**viscera** . . . . . . . . . . .internal organs located inside the body cavity

# N. Quiz Answers

| | | | | | |
|---|---|---|---|---|---|
| 1. b | 16. d | 31. a | 46. c | 61. d | 76. e |
| 2. c | 17. d | 32. c | 47. b | 62. a | 77. d |
| 3. a | 18. e | 33. c | 48. e | 63. d | 78. b |
| 4. e | 19. e | 34. e | 49. d | 64. d | 79. d |
| 5. a | 20. e | 35. e | 50. e | 65. a | 80. b |
| 6. c | 21. e | 36. a | 51. a | 66. e | 81. e |
| 7. b | 22. e | 37. e | 52. c | 67. e | 82. a |
| 8. e | 23. a | 38. a | 53. d | 68. b | 83. c |
| 9. e | 24. d | 39. e | 54. free | 69. c | 84. d |
| 10. e | 25. d | 40. d | 55. b | 70. b | 85. e |
| 11. a | 26. b | 41. c | 56. c | 71. d | 86. e |
| 12. b | 27. c | 42. e | 57. e | 72. b | 87. b |
| 13. c | 28. c | 43. d | 58. c | 73. e | 88. d |
| 14. b | 29. e | 44. c | 59. b | 74. d | 89. a |
| 15. e | 30. b | 45. a | 60. e | 75. e | 90. e |

**Fill in the number of *your* correct answers.** _____

# O. Main Menu for CD ROM

 CD-ROM icon indicates supplemental audio-visual materials that can be seen on the CD.

1. **Scrubbing**

2. **Gowning and Gloving**

3. **Surgical Instruments**
   a. Scalpel
   b. Tissue Scissors
   c. Forceps
   d. Hooks
   e. Retractor
   f. Needle Driver
   g. Hemostat
   h. Cautery
   i. Suture Scissors
   j. Towel Clips
   k. Staple Gun

4. **Knot Tying**
   a. Two-Hand Tie
      1. Square Knot
      2. Surgeon's Knot
   b. Instrument Tie
      1. Surgeon's Knot
      2. Comparison of Square Knot and Surgeon's Knot

# O. Main Menu for CD ROM

5. **Lab Preparation (Pigs' Feet)**

6. **Lab Exercises (Surgical Techniques)**

   a. Instructions and Directions

      1. Making an Incision

      2. Undermining

      3. Principles of Halving

   b. Closing of Skin Suture Techniques

      1. Simple Interrupted Suture

      2. Vertical Mattress

      3. Horizontal Mattress

      4. Running Closure

      5. Running-Lock Closure

      6. Running Intracuticular Closure

      7. Staple Closure

   c. Skin Flaps

      1. Fusiform Excision

      2. Advancement Flap

      3. Rotation Flap

      4. Z-plasty

7. **Quiz**

   a. All the Questions with Answers

   b. 25 Randomized Questions without Answers

# P. Notes from CD

# P. Notes from CD

# Q. Acknowledgments

*Special appreciation to our medical students for evaluating this work; to the creative production team at Mayo, Thomas E. Bibby, Melissa C. Freetly, David M. Jorgenson, Joseph M. Kane, Mark J. McGlinch, and Kurt J. Simon; to the artists, David A. Factor, M. Alice McKinney, and James D. Postier; to our loyal and professional operating room staff, Ann D. Archer, James D. Clark, Linda A. Fenske, Barbara C. Griffith, Karman L. McGill, Barbara K. Pehler-Williams, and Denise K. Webbles; to our secretaries, Michelle T. Franke and Brenda J. Prondzinski; and to Matthew A. Kienstra, M.D., for all their superior help and constructive criticisms which made this work the quality that it is today; finally, a very special thank you in grateful appreciation to our chair, Thomas J. McDonald, M.D., for his more than generous support of this project.*

# R. Instructions for CD ROM Installation

### To install Basic Surgical Skills

Note: If the program is installed on your hard drive, the CD must be in the drive when running the program

#### *Windows 95/98/NT*

1. Insert the Basic Surgical Skills CD ROM  in your CD-ROM drive.
2. After Basic Surgical Skills starts, quit the program.
3. Go to your computer **Start** menu on the task bar.  Select **Run**.
4. Type D:\setup.exe  (or E:\setup.exe if your CD Drive is E: ) and press **Enter.**
5. Follow the on-screen instructions.
6. The installation program will make a Surgical Skills item in your **Programs** menu

#### *Macintosh*

1. Insert the Basic Surgical Skills CD ROM in your CD-ROM drive.
2. Create a folder on your hard drive named "Basic Surgical Skills"
3. Copy the following items to the new folder you just created.
   Surgical Skills
   Xtras folder
   QuickTime Overlay
4. Double-click **Surgical Skills** icon to start the program.

#### *To install QuickTime 4.0*  (Macintosh only)
Macintosh
1. Insert the "Basic Surgical Skills" CD ROM in your CD-ROM drive.
2. Open **QuickTime Installer** folder.
3. Double-click **Installer**.

# S. Operating CD ROM

## To run the program from the CD ROM

### Windows 95/98/NT

1. Insert the Basic Surgical Skills CD ROM in your CD ROM drive.

2. If Basic Surgical Skills does not begin automatically, go to your computer **Start** menu on the task bar. Select **Run**.

3. Type D:\SurgicalSkills.exe (or F urgicalSkills.exe if your CD Drive is E:) and press ter.

### Macintosh

1. Insert the Basic Surgical      D ROM in your CD ROM drive.

2. Double-click the **Surgical Skills** icon.

### Minimum System Requirements

#### Windows 95/98/NT

| | |
|---|---|
| CD-ROM drive: | 4x speed |
| Computer Processor: | 486/90 or faster processor |
| Memory: | 16 MB of RAM |
| Operation System: | Windows 95, Windows 98, or Windows NT 3.51 or 4.0 |
| Hard Disk space: | 15MB of disk space |
| Video: | Compatible SGVA Card |
| Sound: | Soundblaster compatible sound card |

Video for Windows

#### Macintosh

Minimum System requirements:

| | |
|---|---|
| CD-ROM drive: | 4x speed |
| Computer Processor: | Power PC 66 |
| Memory: | 12 MB of RAM |
| Operation System: | System 7.51 |
| Hard Disk space: | 15MB of disk space |
| Video: | Supports thousands/millions of colors |

QuickTime 2 or better